Hospital Human Resource Management

Hospital Human Resource Management

C. Charles

ANMOL PUBLICATIONS PVT. LTD.
NEW DELHI - 110 002 (INDIA)

ANMOL PUBLICATIONS PVT. LTD.
H.O.: 4374/4B, Ansari Road, Darya Ganj
New Delhi-110 002 (India)
Ph.: 23278000, 23261597
B.O.: 1015, Ist Main Road, BSK IIIrd Stage
IIIrd Phase, IIIrd Block
Bangalore - 560 085 (Karnataka)
Ph: 080-41723429, Tel/Fax: 080-2672 3604
Visit us at: www.anmolpublications.com

Hospital Human Resource Management

First Published, 2008

ISBN 978-81-261-3289-8

PRINTED IN INDIA

Printed at Mehra Offset Press, Delhi.

Contents

Preface

This publication entitled "Hospital Human Resource Management" is published specifically to clarify the human resource management aspects of hospital business and healthcare management in the modern age. The focus lies on key issues, including human skills in handling medical technologies, patient care and medical treatments.

Hospital HRM is created to serve the employees of the hospitals. It provides support to the institution through the departments of benefits, the child care center, compensation, development and training, the employee assistance program, employee relations, employment, and temporary services.

This publication entitled "Hospital Human Resource Management" can be used as a reference book for current opinion and the latest developments in the field of hospital human resource management and their utilities in areas, such as, handling of cardiovascular equipment and devices; cleaning and disinfections management; communications and telemedicine; critical care; diagnostics and analysis; facilities management; furniture and fittings; healthcare courses, training and events; healthcare informatics; hospital security systems; implants and fixation devices; handling of laboratory equipment; handling of medical and surgical disposables; medical clothing; medical imaging and diagnostics; patient monitoring; pharmaceuticals and medicines; rehabilitation and mobility; respiratory care and anesthesiology; sterilization; handling of surgical and electro-surgical equipment; and wound-care and dressings. This book "Hospital Human Resource Management" is very useful and reader friendly.

—Editor

1

Introduction to Hospital Human Resource Management

HEALTH SERVICE DELIVERY

Health Workforce Challenges: Lessons from Country Experiences

This report, written for the High Level Forum on Health MDGs, outlines the looming crisis in human resources for health (HRH) confronting most countries in sub-Saharan Africa, and suggests concrete actions that can be taken to avert this crisis. The authors outline three dimensions of the crisis. Firstly, there is an absolute shortage of health workers in some countries. Secondly, human resources are unevenly distributed. Finally, the productivity of human resources is low. The authors argue that these issues are related. For example, the HIV and AIDS epidemic creates new burdens on the health workforce, while at the same time reducing its numbers and productivity. Poor people—in both developed and developing countries—experience more ill health and shorter life spans than their richer fellow citizens. Although people's health is influenced by a wide range of socio-economic and lifestyle factors, access to high quality and affordable health care and public health services makes a critical contribution to health status. Health services are failing poor people—with lower rates of child immunisation, skilled attendance at child birth, and TB and malaria treatment. It's also true that richer groups tend to benefit more from public sector subsidies to health care-hospitals in urban centres often receive disproportionate funds compared with primary care in poor rural areas. And in most poor countries which lack formal taxation and insurance systems, out-of-pocket payments are paid to both private and public providers, consume household income and assets, and contribute to impoverishment. Improving service delivery to the poor involves all the major stakeholders in the health system—the policymakers in ministries of health, finance, and public administration, health service managers and workers, public and private providers and clients and communities themselves. Better access depends on a wide range of factors—on health policies, strategy and plans that prioritise health needs and set out revenue sources and resource requirements (including mechanisms to address inequalities), on motivated and properly trained and remunerated health workers, on infrastructure, drugs and equipment, on good referral links and communication, and – last but not least—on well-informed clients and their representative bodies.

Contracting

In efforts to achieve better performance and greater accountability in the public sector, service providers are being given increasing autonomy. To enable this to work, service provider's inputs and outputs are increasingly specified and agreed through a form of contract or agreement that seeks to protect the public interest. This is particularly important when public finance is being directed to private (non-profit and for-profit) service providers to supply public services. Contracting deals with the various ways in which this can be done, and the problems encountered in practice.

— Contracting and performance management in the health sector: a guide for low and middle income countries

— Contracting for primary health services: evidence on its effects and a framework for evaluation

Private Sector

In all low income countries, private sector health care providers (broadly defined to embrace both for profit and not-for-profit, formal and informal) play a very significant role in service delivery. There is evidence of both positive and negative experiences, but research is generally scarcer than with the public sector, and public policy also tends to neglect this area. Poor people are spending an increasing proportion of their resources on private health care and, in many instances, do not get a 'good bargain' in terms of the health benefits. To achieve both health and poverty development goals, it is therefore imperative that national public health policies and programmes evolve to embrace both the private, as well as the public, sectors, where this has not already happened.

Health Services Management

The rapidly changing and increasingly complex health services industry poses significant challenges for health services management, responsible for planning, directing, coordinating and supervising the delivery of healthcare. Improving service delivery and ensuring better access is complicated by increasing demand due to technological advance, consumer demand, and changes in demography and epidemiology. Health policies, strategies and plans must address both supply and demand side issues to ensure the most efficient management of resources while improving quality and effectiveness. To do this, health services management has to lead the transformation of services at the same time as achieving cost containment and effective performance.

Quality Improvements

Ensuring high quality medical care is a challenge to any health system. If clinical practice is to be effective, diagnosis and treatments should be evidence based, using clinical guidelines; treatment protocols should be cost effective. This in turn will depend on the provision of high quality drugs, which will require transparent systems for drug registration, quality standards, and regulated supply. Health care staff should receive appropriate training, which should be accredited against agreed standards. All should be licensed by professional or governmental bodies, and all training should be ongoing—"professional development". All aspects of health care delivery should be accredited and monitored ("audited") against agreed standards, and clinicians should be answerable for their practice ("clinical governance"). All aspects of quality in health service delivery depend on effective management.

Human Resources

The skills and motivation of the workforce are crucial to health system performance and to the achievement of the Millennium Development Goals. It is therefore essential that the skills and motivation of staff are addressed. Low staff morale, poor health infrastructure and working environments, low pay (contributing to labour migration), and HIV/AIDS widening the gap between staff availability and demand are typical in the public health system. Whilst significant attention has been paid to the development of health strategies and policies, and the financial consequences of those policies, virtually nothing in comparison has been done to address the human resource implications of achieving those policies.

Essential Drugs Management

Viable pharmaceutical services are a core component of functioning health services and therefore of the success of all health strategies. Medicines are central to combating HIV and AIDS, tuberculosis, malaria, and other communicable diseases, and the majority of non-communicable diseases.Since 2003, poor countries are able to import cheaper generic medicines made under compulsory licensing if they are unable to manufacture the drugs themselves; this resulted from the WTO's revision of the 2001 Doha TRIPS (intellectual property) and public health agreement. However, the efficient management of medicines is notoriously difficult, and drug supply fails for many reasons. The WHO has developed a framework for collective action to ensure equitable access to essential drugs. This framework includes rational selection, affordable prices, sustainable financing and a reliable health and supply system. The following list of resources has been chosen to help those with a professional need to develop this aspect of their work using relevant, good quality information. The list connects with WHO's work on essential drugs, and many of the references are documents produced by the Essential Drugs and Medicines Policy Department—generally accepted as the global reference point for best practice on this subject.

SAFETY AND HEALTH TRAINING

Procedures

Safety and health training plans should be developed in conjunction with the annual Performance Appraisal Process. All safety and health training will be reflected in the employee's annual Individual Development Plan. Completion of all formal training will also be documented using Form SF-182, Request, Authorization, Agreement and Certificate of Training.

Purpose

Safety and health training is an integral part of the APHIS Safety and Health Programme. Compliance with training requirements outlined in this section will greatly enhance the ability of supervisors, managers, and employees to fulfill the objectives of the Safety and Health Programme. Training requirements specified in this Chapter are mandatory, and meet the minimum legal requirements of OSHA.

Specific Training Requirements

There are some specific training requirements for certain categories of employees and certain types of work functions. These requirements are summarized below and represent the minimum Agency requirements. Organizational heads may require additional training as deemed necessary for any category of employee or type of work functions. Training Requirements for CDSHOs. CDSHOs have been divided into four categories as listed below. The minimum training programme requirement, for the Regional CDSHOs are especially important because these individuals assist in the training of other safety and health officers, employees, and supervisors in their respective regions. The minimum training requirements are as follows:

Regional CDSHOs. Training or orientation in the following: APHIS Safety and Health Programme, accident investigation and reporting procedures, collateral duty safety and health responsibilities, effective safety and health councils, hazardous chemicals safety, inspection procedures, selection and use of respirators, and the APHIS Annual National Safety and Health Symposium.

Latin American CDSHOs. Training or orientation in the following: APHIS Safety and Health Programme, accident investigation and reporting procedures, and the APHIS

Annual Safety and Health Symposium.

Laboratory CDSHOs. Specialized training or orientation in the following: Collateral duty safety and health responsibilities, hazardous chemicals safety, inspection procedures, effective safety and health councils, and the selection and use of respirators.

Programme CDSHOs, e.g., Tick Force. Specialized training or orientation in the following: Collateral duty safety and health responsibilities, effective safety and health councils, selection and use of respirators, and pesticide application.

These training requirements are listed by priority of importance. Training will commence within 3 months of assignment to duties, and 2 courses should be completed each year until all requirements are met.

First Aid Training. The ready access to a professionally staffed medical facility will be the primary determinant in whether an employee within a unit is required to take first aid training. The supervisor will determine who and how many employees are to take the training if a professionally staffed medical facility is not readily accessible. However, supervisors should promote first aid training to all employees. Employees granted approval by supervisors to take first aid training will not be charged leave to attend classes. The names of those employees trained to render first aid will be known to all other employees within the unit. Supervisors will ensure that employees who work alone are capable of handling emergencies expected in their working environment.

Standard first aid training must be American Red Cross (ARC) or equivalent. Employees successfully completing the course will be issued certification cards, which are valid for 3 years.

Cardiopulmonary Resuscitation (CPR) Training. The requirements regarding first aid training are also applicable to CPR. CPR training and certification is provided nationally through the Red Cross and the American Heart Association. Employees granted approval by supervisors to take CPR training will not be charged leave to attend classes. CPR training is valid for 1 year. In addition to the minimum requirements, supervisors should promote CPR training for all employees regardless of access to medical facilities or job hazards.

General Training Requirements

General safety and health training requirements are summarized below. It is the responsibility of the individual supervisor and the appropriate Collateral Duty Safety and Health Officer (CDSHO) to ensure that training requirements are fulfilled. Top Management Officials. Orientation with: Section 19 of the Occupational Safety and Health Act, Executive Order 12196, 29 CFR Part 1960, and the APHIS Safety and Health Manual. Supervisors. Orientation with: Section 19 of the Occupational Safety and Health Act, Executive Order 12196, 29 CFR Part 1960, the APHIS Safety and Health Manual, and OSHA standards applicable to the assigned workplace and operations under their control. Employees. Specialized training/orientation appropriate to the work performed by the employee, e.g., printing office, pesticide operations, laboratory work, etc., which includes safety and health requirements of the job; defensive driving when appropriate; rights and responsibilities associated with the APHIS Safety and Health Programme. Employee Representatives. Training in the recognition of hazardous conditions and work practices commensurate with the scope of assigned responsibilities concerning the APHIS Safety and Health Programme.

EMPLOYEE INFORMATION AND TRAINING

Training

Each laboratory supervisor is responsible for ensuring that laboratory employees are provided with training about the hazards of chemicals present in their laboratory work area, and methods to control exposure to such chemicals. Such training must be provided at the time of an employee's initial assignment to a work area where hazardous chemicals are present and prior to assignments involving new potential exposure situations. Refresher training must be provided annually.

Colleges and non-academic departments that engage in the laboratory use of hazardous chemicals are responsible for identifying employees who require training and for developing and delivering training programmes for such employees. DEHS offers training on the third Thursday of each month that covers general laboratory safety issues, hazardous waste management, and biohazardous materials handling. Departments are welcome to send employees to this 'base' training at no charge. However, laboratory supervisors must provide additional training on laboratory-specific hazards to ensure all the OSHA-required training topics have been adequately addressed. Call DEHS at 626-6002 to register trainees.

Employee training programmes will include, at a minimum, the following subjects:

— Methods of detecting the presence of hazardous chemicals;

— Method include visual observation, odor, real-time air monitoring, time-weighted air sampling, etc.).

— Basic toxicological principles;

- Principles include toxicity, hazard, exposure, routes of entry, acute and chronic effects, dose-response relationship, LD50, threshold limit values and permissible exposure limits, exposure time, and health hazards related to classes of chemicals.
- Prudent laboratory practices;
- Prudent laboratory practices include general techniques designed to reduce personal exposure and to control physical hazards, as well as specific protective mechanisms and warning systems used in individual laboratories. Appropriate use of fume hoods is to be specifically addressed.
- Description of available chemical information;
- Container labels, Material Safety Data Sheets, etc.
- Emergency response actions appropriate to individual laboratories;
- Lists of emergency phone numbers, location of fire extinguishers, deluge showers, eyewashes, etc.
- Applicable details of the departmental Laboratory Safety Plan;
- Details should include general and laboratory-specific Standard Operating Procedures.
- An introduction to the Hazardous Chemical Waste Management guidebook; and
- The script for the video Laboratory Chemicals and Your Health.

Information

It is essential that laboratory employees have access to information on the hazards of chemicals and procedures for working safely. Supervisors must ensure that laboratory employees are informed about and have access to the following information sources:

The University of Minnesota's Laboratory Safety Plan

This generic LSP is available to all employees on the Department of Environmental Health and Safety's web site (www.dehs.umn.edu) and in the Learning Resource Centers of the various campus libraries. Individual department Laboratory Safety Plans are available within those departments.

The Contents of the OSHA Laboratory Safety Standard

"Occupational Exposure to Hazardous Chemicals in Laboratories" and its appendices (29 CFR 1910.1450). A copy of this federal standard can be found in Appendix A of this Laboratory Safety Plan.

The Permissible Exposure Limits (PELs)

PELs for OSHA regulated substances can be found in Appendix B. Also included in Appendix B are the ACGIH Threshold Limit Value (TLV) list, a list of OSHA health hazard definitions, lists of "select carcinogens" and reproductive toxins, and chemicals having a high degree of acute toxicity.

Laboratory Chemical Safety Summaries (LCSSs) are included on pages 235-413 of the 1995 edition of Prudent Practices. LCSSs are similar to Material Safety Data Sheets (MSDS), but are tailored to the hazards of laboratory use of those chemicals. The LCSSs include toxicity information, and signs and symptoms of exposure to the chemicals.

Material Safety Data Sheets (MSDSs)

MSDSs are available online through links from the Department of Environmental Health and Safety's web site. Hard copies of MSDS for many laboratory chemicals are also available from DEHS or departmental safety offices. Individual researchers are encouraged to keep hard copies in an easily accessible location for materials that are used in large quantities, which are used frequently, or which are particularly toxic.

Information on chemical waste disposal and spill response

The University of Minnesota guidebook, Hazardous Chemical Waste Management 5rd edition provides detailed information on proper waste handling procedures.

CREW RESOURCE MANAGEMENT AND ITS APPLICATIONS IN MEDICINE

Patient care, like other technically complex and high risk fields, is an interdependent process carried out by teams of individuals with advanced technical training who have varying roles and decision-making responsibilities. While technical training assures proficiency at specific tasks, it does not address the potential for errors created by communicating and decision making in dynamic environments. Experts in aviation have developed safety training focused on effective team management, known as Crew Resource Management (CRM). Improvements in the safety record of commercial aviation may be due, in part, to this training. Over the past 10 years, lessons from aviation's approach to team training have been applied to patient safety, notably in intensive care unit (ICU) and anesthesia training. This chapter reviews the literature on Crew Resource Management, also known as Cockpit Resource Management, and describes adaptations of this training framework to medicine.

Prevalence and Severity of the Target Safety Problem

The field of aviation has a substantial history of collecting and analysing safety-related data. Historically, human error has caused or contributed to over 50% of aviation accidents. In an analysis of 35,000 reports of incidents over 7.5 years, almost 50% resulted from a flight crew error, and an additional 35% were attributed to air traffic controller error. Root cause analyses by safety experts have found that errors frequently occur because flight crews fail to effectively manage the resources available to them (e.g., fail to verify information when uncertain about it, fail to plan for contingencies). Naval aviation reports provide similar results, with one study reporting 59% of "Class A mishaps" (serious consequences including fatality, destroyed aircraft, and major injury) attributed to some degree to aircrew factors. These and similar analyses have catalyzed tailored prevention strategies including CRM for commercial aviation, and "aircrew coordination training" (ACT) for Naval aviators.

Practice Description

Crew Resource Management in Aviation

Crew Resource Management has been widely used to improve the operation of flight crews. The concept originated in 1979, in response to a NASA workshop that examined the role that human error plays in air crashes. CRM emphasizes the role of human factors in high-stress, high-risk environments. John K. Lauber, a psychologist member of the National Transportation Safety Board, defined CRM as "using all available sources—information, equipment, and people—to achieve safe and efficient flight operations." CRM encompasses team training, as well as simulation (also referred to as *Line-Oriented Flight Training*, or LOFT), interactive group debriefings, and measurement and improvement of aircrew performance. There is no universal CRM training programme. The Federal Aviation Administration (FAA) allows air carriers to customize their CRM programmes to best suit the needs of individual organisations. Therefore, training programmes vary somewhat from carrier to carrier, making it difficult to describe operational components. Furthermore, these programmes continue to evolve as aviation technology changes and more is learned about group dynamics. One CRM model focuses on the elements of human effectiveness. The 3 primary components of effective crew management are safety, efficiency, and morale. Specific factors related to aircrew performance are categorized, and serve as the basis for training and research. These factors include materials, organisation, individual, and group process variables associated with performance. Examples of outcomes that result from these input variables are safety, efficiency, and customer satisfaction. Subsequently, Helmreich and colleagues proposed a modified conceptual framework for CRM, termed the "Error Troika," to display a hierarchy of 3 error countermeasures.

At the first level, CRM includes training on how to avoid errors. At the second level, potential errors are "trapped" before they are committed. At the third level, mitigation of error consequences occurs. From a practical standpoint, CRM programmes typically include educating crews about the limitations of human performance. Trainees develop an understanding of cognitive errors, and how stressors (such as fatigue, emergencies, and work overload) contribute to the occurrence of errors. Multi-day CRM training programmes typically require participants to assess personal and peer behaviour. Operational concepts stressed include inquiry, seeking relevant operational information, advocacy, communicating proposed actions, conflict resolution and decision making.

Practice Description

Crew Resource Management in Healthcare Settings

As with aviation, the medical application of CRM has required tailoring of training approaches to mirror the areas in which human factors contribute to mishaps. In anesthesiology 65-70% of safety problems (accidents or incidents) have been attributed at least in part to human error. In response, several anesthesiologists from the VA Palo Alto Health Care System and Stanford University, with funding from the Anesthesia Patient Safety Foundation, developed *Anesthesia Crisis Resource Management* (ACRM), modeled on CRM. The original demonstration courses consisted of didactic instruction, videotape of a reenactment of an aviation disaster, videotape of an actual anesthetic mishap, simulation training and a debriefing session. Ongoing courses include the use of a textbook that catalogues 83 critical events (e.g., acute hemorrhage, bronchospasm, seizures), and approaches to managing them. Currently, there are 3 ACRM courses offering progressively more challenging material, a Working Group on Crisis Management Training in Health Care formed by the developers of ACRM that has initiated formal ACRM instructor training, and thoughtful consideration of pragmatic approaches to evaluating ACRM.

Helmreich and Schaefer have also advanced CRM theory in the operating room environment by adapting their model of team performance. This framework describes the team performance inputs that are critical to essential team functions that in turn lead to desired outcomes (defined as patient well-being). Examples of inputs include individual aptitudes, physical environment, and culture (professional, organisational, and national). Performance functions consist of team formation and management, surgical procedures, communications, decision processes, and situational awareness. Another application of CRM to the health environment is the *MedTeams behaviour-based teamwork system*, developed by Dynamics Research Corporation, and sponsored by the Army Research Laboratory. It aims to adapt research in team performance and training from military helicopter aviation to emergency medicine. Thus far, specific applications have been developed for Emergency Department care and labor and delivery units. The system is implemented through courses and assessment tools. The Emergency Team Coordination Course (ETCC) includes 5 team dimensions or goals (i.e., maintain team structure and climate, facilitate planning and problem-solving, enhance communication among team members, facilitate workload management, improve team-building skills). Each goal is tied to specific teamwork tasks. For example, tasks for the first goal (maintain team structure and climate) include "establish team leader," "form the team," "set team goals," and "assign roles and responsibilities." Like the CRM approach to the "Error Troika," the MedTeams approach is based on avoiding errors, trapping them as they occur, and mitigating the consequences of actual errors. Principles underlying the MedTeams approach include:

— Team responsibility for patients.
— A belief in clinician fallibility.
— Peer monitoring.
— Team member awareness of patient status, team member status and institutional resources.

Peer monitoring is a fundamental component of the MedTeams system, as well as a feature of the ACRM and aviation field's CRM approaches. Along with his or her clinical responsibilities, each team member undertakes the intermittent process of peer monitoring or "check" actions, engaging in this check cycle as frequently as possible. The teamwork check cycle begins with each team member monitoring his or her own situation awareness and cross-monitoring the actions of other teammates. If during the monitoring mode the *monitoring* teammate observes a suspected error in progress, that individual intervenes with a direct question or offer of information. The erring teammate may then acknowledge the lapse, correct it and continue working. Alternatively, the *monitoring* teammate may have lost situation awareness. The non-erring *monitored* colleague can then provide feedback to correct the peer's situation awareness. If team members are in strong disagreement about how patient care should proceed, advocacy, assertion and perhaps third-party involvement may be used to resolve the situation.

Over time, the check cycle becomes habitual, resulting in hundreds of team checks daily, all with the potential to break the error chain. Recently, ACRM has been extended to a full-day course on neonatal resuscitation training for neonatologists and pediatricians. Called "NeoSim", the course combines traditional training methods with reviews of literature and didactic instruction with simulation. Debriefing follows, using videotape of the simulation. As with the other examples, the emphasis of teaching behavioural teamwork skills along with technical content is the hallmark of CRM interventions in healthcare.

Applications of CRM Principles in Medicine

The Sexton study and other analyses suggest that safety-related behaviours that have been applied and studied extensively in the aviation industry may also be relevant in healthcare. We identified CRM applications in several dynamic decision-making healthcare environments: the operating room, labor and delivery, and the emergency room. In addition, Gaba has noted that some other domains (e.g., cardiac arrest response teams) that have active simulation training are currently incorporating a broader range of CRM-like training methods.

Study Design and Outcomes

Measures

Although the most obvious and meaningful measure of CRM effectiveness would appear to be airline accident or "near miss" rates, these objective measures have not been used in commercial aviation studies. Helmreich suggests that it is not possible to use these measures, because accident rates are very low and "near misses" are voluntarily reported. Furthermore, the content and structure of CRM training programmes are variable. In response, researchers have developed tools that assess the effectiveness of CRM in other ways. These tools include attitudinal surveys and peer performance rating questionnaires, including the NASA/ University of Texas Line/LOS Checklist (LINE/LOS Checklist), the Cockpit Management Attitudes Questionnaire (CMAQ), and the Flight Management Attitudes Questionnaire (FMAQ).

The LINE/LOS Checklist is used to rate crew performance on critical behaviours during specific segments of flight (e.g., not rushing through briefing period, exhibiting high levels of vigilance in both high and low workload conditions, etc). Ratings on each behavioural element (i.e., model for teamwork) range across 4 levels from poor to outstanding. In contrast, CMAQ is used to evaluate the attitudes of crewmembers within and between organisations, pre- and/ or post-CRM training.

Results are intended to serve as a proxy for measuring crew process and performance. The instrument has been validated by comparing self-reported attitudes with performance ratings made by experienced Check Airmen, experts trained in peer evaluation. The FMAQ is a revised version of the CMAQ that was developed by Helmreich and colleagues in response to attitudinal differences observed in flight crews from different countries. Observation of crew performance in simulated flights has also been used.

Representative Studies

Several studies have utilized proxy tools to test the effectiveness of CRM. One study by Helmreich and colleagues consisted of an assessment of the attitudes before versus after CRM training (pre-test versus post-test). Crew behaviours were noted by a trained observer using the NASA/University of Texas Line/LOS Checklist. More than 2000 line flights and LOFT sessions were included in the analysis. Overall performance of crews was classified as "below average," "average," or "above average" by Check Airmen and LOFT instructors.

As a result of the CRM training, the percentage of crews rated as "above average" increased while the percent rated "below average" decreased. Performance ratings differed between fleets and airlines. Superior pilots also shared many common attitudes, (for example, they were aware of their personal limitations and diminished decision-making capacity during emergencies). In addition, they encouraged crewmembers to question their decisions and actions, were sensitive to the personal problems of other crewmembers, and recognized the need to verbalize plans and to train other crewmembers. A second study by Barker and colleagues compared the effectiveness of 17 CRM-trained flight crews on military mission simulators, divided according to whether they were "fixed" or "formed" crews. Nine of the crews were defined as "fixed" since they had flown together for six months or longer; the remaining 8 were "formed," as they had flown together for less than 6 months. Each crew was asked to participate in a simulated mission. The first leg of the mission was programmed to be problem-free, but the second leg required crews to address a safety issue. As with the earlier study, crew behaviours were observed using the NASA/University of Texas Line/LOS Checklist. Surprisingly, the formed crews committed fewer minor errors, but the number of major errors did not differ significantly between the groups. The authors concluded that formed crews may experience less ineffective coordination than fixed crews, as the latter might be more complacent from the routine of working together, but that further research was needed.

A third study evaluated rates of naval aviation mishaps, and the role of CRM failures. While the study primarily compared crew performance in 2 types of equipment, the aircrew performance deficits were also compared with those seen during an earlier time period, prior to implementation of aircrew coordinating training (ACT) programmes (the specific form of CRM used). Analysis of data from the post-ACT implementation period across the fleet revealed that 70% of human error mishaps were connected with aircrew factors, and that 56% of these resulted from at least one CRM failure. The authors noted that these percentages were similar to those reported in a separate study prior to ACT implementation. Because of a lack of controls or adjustments for potential confounders, no conclusions about effectiveness of the ACT programme can be drawn.

Comparison to Medicine

Sexton and colleagues compared flight crews with operating room personnel on several measures, including attitudes toward teamwork. The study included more than 30,000 cockpit crew members (captains, first officers, and second officers) and 1033 operating room personnel (attending surgeons, attending anesthesiologists, surgical residents, anesthesia residents, surgical nurses, anesthesia nurses). Data from the crew members were obtained from previous administrations of the CMAQ and FMAQ to major airlines around the world (over a 15-year period). The operating room participants were mailed an analogous questionnaire (CMAQ modified), administered over a period of 3 years at 12 teaching and non-teaching hospitals in the United States and abroad (Italy, Germany, Switzerland, and Israel). The level of teamwork perceived by attending surgeons compared with other operating room staff differed markedly. A majority of surgical residents (73%) and attending surgeons (64%) reported high levels of teamwork, but only 39% of attending anesthesiologists, 28% of surgical nurses, 25% of anesthesia nurses, and 10% of anesthesia residents reported high levels of teamwork.

A bare majority (55%) of attending surgeons rejected steep hierarchies (determined by whether they thought junior team members should question the decisions of senior team members). In contrast, 94% of airline crew members preferred flat hierarchies. It was also noted that medical participants were far more likely to agree with the statement "Even when fatigued, I perform effectively during critical times." Seventy percent of attending surgeons agreed with this statement, as well as 56% of surgical residents, 60% of surgical nurses, 57% of anesthesia residents, 55% of anesthesia nurses, and 47% of attending anesthesiologists. In contrast, 26% of pilots agreed with this statement.

Evidence for Effectiveness of the Practice

The most thoroughly studied of the medical CRM applications is ACRM, although as with the aviation examples, rigorous evaluations are challenging to design. Few studies utilize a control group, although researchers have reported assessment methods for determining both technical and behavioural performance from simulator videotapes. A before-after ACRM training analysis (Level 3 Study Design) of trainees' knowledge-base (Level 3 Outcome) for crisis yielded mixed results. The average score on the post-test was significantly greater than the pre-test for one trainee class, composed mostly of residents. For the other class of experienced anesthesiologists, the test scores did not change and were at the same level as the post-test scores of class of residents.

Subjective data evaluating the course indicated that trainees "uniformly felt that the ACRM course was an intense, superior form of training related to an important, but inadequately taught, component of anesthesia practice." Another study of ACRM at Harvard also found that participants rated the course favourably, with over 80% responding that they felt the course should be taken every 24 months or less. As with aviation, the incremental value of this form of training is difficult to link to improvements in teamwork performance and better safety records. At the time of this literature assessment, there were no published data to describe the effects on medical error rates of the MedTeams approach. The NeoSim course participants provided positive responses to open-ended questions about their satisfaction with the course.

Costs and Implementation

Helmreich has noted some of the limitations associated with CRM. At this time, the evidence connecting CRM approaches to improving patient safety does not exist, notwithstanding the face validity of the approach. Nevertheless, a long history of variants of the approach offers healthcare a reasonable foundation from which to draw practical and evidenced-based resources for further development and adaptation of CRM, as well as measurement methods to ascertain its effectiveness. At a minimum, implementation of the CRM approach in healthcare settings requires customisation of tools and techniques for each specific care venue, as is illustrated by adaptations implemented thus far. This customisation comes at considerable cost and cannot be expected to immediately reap safety benefits. At the time of this review, approximate costs for implementing the MedTeams system ranged from $15,000-$35,000, with additional costs for ongoing activities (such as continuing education) that ranged from $8,000-$20,000 (R. Simon, personal communication, April 2001). Similarly, marginal costs for CRM-like training based on the ACRM experience are estimated at $800 to $2,000 per participant per day (D.M. Gaba, personal communication, June 2001).

LABORATORY SAFETY PLAN: PERSONNEL

RSO's – note and delete: Compliance with the Laboratory Safety Standard is a shared responsibility. In Subsection B, note whether the LSP covers an entire college, a department or a specific laboratory only. Provide the name of the Research Safety Officer, and describe the RSOs assigned responsibilities. As noted in this study, includes typical responsibilities of a departmental RSO. Some of these responsibilities may be delegated to safety committee members (if a safety committee exists), or additional duties may be added at the discretion of the department. In Subsection C, note whether or not a safety committee has been formed, and if so, what its responsibilities are. The following individuals and groups have responsibilities for implementation of various aspects of the University of Minnesota's Laboratory Safety Plan.

College or Departmental Safety Committee

The designation of a safety committee to assist the safety officer in his/her required duties is strongly encouraged. Names of the safety committee members should be listed in this paragraph.

ADDITIONAL EMPLOYEE PROTECTION FOR WORK WITH PARTICULARLY HAZARDOUS SUBSTANCES

RSO's – note and delete: Like Section 6, this Section also requires action. Again, the PIs in the department must consider the toxicity of the chemicals used and the hazards of each procedure, and decide whether the procedure requires the use of additional protective measures. Chemicals listed could be considered for additional protective measures. The additional protective measures should be incorporated in the Standard Operating Procedure. Each PI should forward a list of these SOPs to the departmental Research Safety Officer for reference in this section of the LSP. If none of the SOPs require additional protective measures, the PI should note this fact and forward a brief explanation to the RSO. EHS staff is available to help PIs evaluate the need for additional protective measures.

Additional employee protection will be considered for work with particularly hazardous substances. These include select carcinogens, reproductive toxins and substances that have a high degree of acute toxicity. These pages may be accessed from DEHS's web site at www.dehs.umn.edu. Also, DEHS has hard copies of the entire 1995 edition available for departmental Research Safety Officers. Laboratory supervisors and principal investigators are responsible for assuring that laboratory procedures involving particularly hazardous chemicals have been evaluated for the level of employee protection required. Specific consideration will be given to the need for inclusion of the following provisions:

1. Planning;
2. Establishment of a designated area;
3. Access control
4. Special precautions such as:

- — use of containment devices such as fume hoods or glove boxes;
- — use of personal protective equipment;
- — isolation of contaminated equipment;
- — practicing good laboratory hygiene; and
- — prudent transportation of very toxic chemicals.

5. Planning for accidents and spills; and
6. Special storage and waste disposal practices.

Occupational Physician

The University of Minnesota's Boynton Health Service provides limited occupational medicine services. The phone number for the Occupational Medicine programme, which covers Research Animal Resources, respiratory protection, and pesticide exposures only, is 612-625-4906. Non hospital employee chemical exposures should go through Boynton's urgent care.

HUMAN FACTORS AND MEDICAL DEVICES

Human factors engineering (HFE), also known as *usability engineering* or *ergonomics*, is the study of how humans interact with machines and complex systems. Through the merging of cognitive psychology, engineering and other disciplines, human factors researchers have detailed numerous principles concerning device and software programme designs that allow for optimal usage. When these principles are violated, improper use of a machine is more likely to result. Specific examples have been detailed during observations of user errors with electronic infusion devices. Medical device misuse is an important cause of medical error, and therefore, incorporating human factors methodology into the design of medical devices has assumed an important role in ensuring patient safety. This study describes the use of HFE principles as a safety practice in the design of medical devices and their evaluation both prior to and after institutional purchase. Next, medical device alarms and the contribution of HFE to alarm improvements will be evaluated. Finally, the chapter reviews the use of preoperative checklist procedures to reduce anesthesia device failures. Human factors engineering is a powerful component in the design of usable, safe medical devices. HFE principles can be incorporated as safety practices that occur at various points during device development and usage.

Industry can use HFE principles at multiple times in the design and developmental cycle of medical devices and software packages. Healthcare institutions can consider results of HFE evaluations when deciding which products to purchase. Finally, HFE principles can also be incorporated into the ongoing evaluation of devices that have already been purchased and are in use. While these practices have high face validity, there has been little formal study of their effectiveness in reducing medical error. They are presented here because they may hold promise if scrutinized rigorously, and to familiarize readers with their potential to reduce medical error.

Design and Developmental Phase

Data collected by the United States Food and Drug Administration (FDA) in the late 1980s demonstrated that almost half of all medical device recalls resulted from design flaws. In 1990, Congress passed the Safe Medical Devices Act, giving the FDA the ability to mandate good manufacturing practices (GMP). These GMP involve design controls for manufacturers that help ensure the use of HFE within medical device design. As described in the Good Manufacturing Practice Regulation, Design Control subsection (Title 21-Section 820.30), these include the use of iterative design and testing during the developmental phase.

The Act requires that designs be "appropriate and address the intended use of the device, including the needs of the user and patient." Multiple human factors techniques, such as user studies, prototype tests, and task/function analysis, are utilized in the development and design process. Manufacturers are required not only to use human factors principles to repeatedly test the product in all phases of design, but also to validate the ultimate device design. Validation entails testing the device, either in an actual clinical situation or a simulation, and documenting that the device conforms to the individual user's needs. Thus, manufacturers are required to apply HFE methods through the multiple phases of device design and development cycles.

Human factors engineering practices for medical device design and evaluation have been well described. In 1993 the Association for the Advancement of Medical Instrumentation and the American National Standards Institute established guidelines for the incorporation of HFE principles into medical device design. This comprehensive document helped direct attention to the problem of poor medical device design and helped establish the design standards necessary to ensure safe medical equipment and thus should stand as the safety benchmark for industry. Only limited data are available concerning the application of HFE principles to medical device design, and most are not published. Nonetheless, the application of human factors principles during a device's design phase has been demonstrated to reduce user error. Patient controlled analgesia (PCA) pumps are a case in point of how HFE principles in product design reduce user error.

User errors associated with poor interface design have been described with PCA pumps. Lin and colleagues investigated whether applying human factors engineering principles to the design of the user interface of a PCA pump could result in fewer dosage errors as well as less time spent programming the device. Information on device usage was obtained through cognitive task analysis. This involved observing and interviewing nurses operating PCA pumps both in the laboratory setting and in the field. Utilizing this feedback, as well as other human factors design principles, a "new" PCA pump interface was designed. Twelve recovery room nurses were required to complete specific tasks with both the standard PCA user interface and the newly designed interface. There were 29 programming errors on the traditional interface and 13 on the redesigned interface (an error reduction of 55%, $p<0.01$). Furthermore, users were able to programme in the necessary orders in 18% less time.

Another example involves the design of an ultrasound machine. In this study, Aucella and colleagues interviewed sonographers, videotaped the ultrasound device being used, and performed usability testing through simulation to collect information regarding the operator-machine interface of the ultrasound machine. After their extensive investigations they implemented over 100 design changes to the console and control panel. Although errors with the machine were not measured, comments collected by the authors from the beta operators of the newly designed device suggested that the resulting machine was much easier to use. There are enormous numbers of medical devices and software being designed and developed. Thus the FDA has initiated several regulatory mechanisms to ensure compliance with these guidelines. Some of the mechanisms include site inspections of manufacturers, review and approval of medical devices before marketing, and review of medical device incident reports. Despite the tremendous amount of effort put forth by the FDA to ensure compliance with the Good Manufacturing Practices Regulation, individual institutions should critically analyse whether a device they intend to purchase meets HFE principles for user-centered design.

FATIGUE, SLEEPINESS, AND MEDICAL ERRORS

Fatigue may contribute to the human error component of medical errors. Hospitals function around the clock, which necessitates shift work for many personnel. Physicians, especially those in training, typically work long hours and are often sleep deprived. Personnel who work during evenings and at night experience disruptions in circadian rhythms, which may aggravate fatigue. Although little research has focused specifically on fatigue in hospital personnel and its relationship to medical error, studies outside the medical field demonstrate the intuitive link between fatigue and degradation in performance and suggest some safety practices that may be adopted in medicine. Although both acute and chronic fatigue may have detrimental effects on the health of medical practitioners, this chapter focuses on fatigue's direct effects on patient safety. We review the literature on problem sleepiness among medical personnel, its impact on performance, and interventions to address sleep deprivation: limiting work hours, changes in shift scheduling, napping, and pharmaceutical aids. Although beyond the scope of this chapter, factors that contribute to fatigue beyond sleepiness, such as job stress and work load, should be considered as part of a multifaceted strategy to combat fatigue. Fatigue and sleepiness may affect patient safety in several ways. Physicians and nurses need good attention, sound judgment, and often quick reaction time, especially in emergency situations.

Whether evaluating an electrocardiogram for signs of myocardial ischemia or monitoring a patient during general anesthesia, degradation of attention, memory, or coordination may affect performance and lead to adverse events. Research suggests that sleep requirements and patterns are idiosyncratic, with wide variation across populations. In order to design interventions that will effectively decrease or prevent these events, it is important to understand the signs, prevalence, and impact of sleep deprivation and problem sleepiness.

Sleep Deprivation

Individuals differ in their optimal sleep requirements. Most sleep experts agree that adults typically need between 6 and 10 hours of sleep per 24-hour period, with most people requiring approximately 8 hours of sleep per day. When adults get less than 5 hours of sleep over a 24-hour period, peak mental abilities begin to decline. For short periods of time (2-3 days), adult who get 4 hours of sleep can function reasonably well, but below peak levels. However, even with sleep deprivation of just a couple of days, slower response times and decreased initiatives are observed. After one night of missed sleep, cognitive performance may decrease 25% from baseline. After the second night of missed sleep, cognitive performance can fall to nearly 40% of baseline. With ongoing sleep deprivation (getting 2 to 3 hours less sleep than optimal), people develop a *sleep debt*. If the sleep debt continues over 5 to 10 days, they are rarely maximally alert and at some point general performance, and particularly cognitive performance, become verifiably worse. Sleep debt also leads to slower response times, altered mood and motivation, and reduced morale and initiative. A meta-analysis of the effect of sleep deprivation on performance by Pilcher et al found that humans who are chronically sleep deprived function at the 9 percentile of non-sleep-deprived subjects. Further, sleep deprivation affected mood more than it did cognitive function; both were more affected than motor function.

Night-Shifts and Shift Rotation

Shift work usually refers to a schedule in which some employees begin work at times other than the morning. In hospitals, up to 35% of nurses may be required to work at times other than the day shift. A report by the Association of Professional Sleep Societies concluded that night-time operators' fatigue contributed to 4 well known disasters: Exxon Valdez, Bhopal, Chernobyl, and Three Mile Island. Fatigue has also been implicated in aircraft accidents and in poor driving and accidents among truck drivers.

It is well documented that shift workers have disturbances in their circadian rhythm, as measured by changes in their melatonin and cortisol levels. Sleep after night work tends to be shorter than sleep after day work, leading to greater cumulative sleep deprivation. Shift workers have poorer quality of sleep, marked by less REM sleep, and are less likely to feel refreshed after awaking. Between 60 and 70 percent of shift workers complain of sleeping difficulties or problem sleepiness. Several surveys of shift workers have found that those who work during night shifts are more likely to report sleepiness at work. Alertness on the job is also affected, with employees showing less alertness during nighttime shifts. In addition, shift workers tend to perform less well on reasoning and non-stimulating tasks than non-shift workers.

Prevalence and Severity

Fatigue and sleep deprivation are common among medical personnel. Long work-hours are a tradition during residency, with most interns and residents working 80 to 100 hours a week, often 36 hours at a time. During these shifts their sleep is limited, and is usually interrupted. In a 1991 national survey, second-year residents reported an average of 37.6 hours as the largest number of hours without sleep during their first postgraduate year and roughly 25% of the residents reported being on call in the hospital over 80 hours per week. A movement in the late 1980s, prompted partly by the death of a young woman, led to regulations in New York State dictating that residents could work a maximum of 80 hours per week, with a maximum of 24 consecutive hours of patient care, and a minimum of 8 hours off duty between shifts. Despite these regulations, unannounced inspections of 12 teaching hospitals in New York State in March 1998 found 37% of all residents worked more than 85 hours per week, 20% of all residents and 60% of surgical residents worked more than 95 hours per week, and 38% of all residents and 67% of all surgical residents worked more than 24 consecutive hours. In 2000, 8% of programmes and institutions reviewed by the Accreditation Council for Graduate Medical Education were cited as being in violation of their work-hour requirements. Work-hour violations were noted in general surgery (35%), pediatrics (16%), internal medicine (10%) and other training programmes as well. Long hours and sleep deprivation continue after residency. Healthcare providers, particularly those still in training or who have recently completed training, occasionally work extra shifts to increase their income ("moonlighting"). One recent survey found that nearly half of all emergency medicine residents moonlight. As many as 65% of internal medicine residents and fellows moonlight and moonlighting is common among other residencies and fellowships. These shifts are often at odd hours, and therefore are disruptive to normal sleep patterns. Among surgical staff, fatigue is common, especially since surgical teams can be involved in long, complicated operative cases that can take 12 to 20 hours at a time.

Multiple studies have documented the impact of fatigue on medical personnel performance. However, these studies have been limited by poor study designs or outcomes that may not correlate well with medical error. One study of nursing fatigue suggests that it may play a role in increased error. Gold and colleagues administered a questionnaire to nurses at a large academic hospital and found that nurses who worked a rotating schedule, when compared with nurses who predominantly worked day shifts, were more likely to fall asleep at work and get less sleep over all, and were nearly twice as likely to report committing a medication error.

Using standardized testing, investigators have found that after a night of call, sleep deprived physicians may have worse language and numeric skills, retention of information, short-term memory, and concentration. Performance on standardized tests may not reflect performance in medical situations. Taffinder et al studied the impact of sleep deprivation on surgical residents previously trained on a simulator and found that after a night without sleep, surgeons were slower and more prone to errors on the simulator than those who had a normal night of sleep. Similarly, Denisco et al studied anesthesia residents after a night of sleep deprivation and found that those who had been on call and were sleep deprived scored less well on simulated critical events. Smith-Coggins et al compared cognitive and motor performance of emergency physicians and found that, as the 24-hour study period progressed, physicians were more likely to make errors during a simulated triage test and while intubating a mannequin. However, other studies have failed to find an effect of sleep deprivation on cognitive performance by resident physicians. Simulators may not reflect actual medical performance.

Though psychomotor performance seems to be affected by sleep deprivation, data are inconsistent as to fatigue's impact on cognitive function and there are inadequate data assessing its impact on clinical performance. Few studies have looked at the impact of fatigue in hospital personnel on adverse events. A retrospective study by Haynes et al of 6371 surgical cases, found that the risk of postoperative complications among patients undergoing surgery was not increased when the surgical resident was sleep deprived. These results may not be surprising for several reasons. First, the authors did not measure the residents' error rate, which may have been higher with sleep deprivation. Second, the study did not measure the role attending physicians or other operating room personnel may have played in averting adverse events when residents erred. The supervisory aspect of system design can (and should) reduce both the frequency of individual mistakes (*error prevention*) and the likelihood of adverse events given that errors are inevitable (*error absorption*). Finally, the rate of adverse events, including those that did not result in operative complications ("near misses"), may have been higher but under reported. Well-designed studies that evaluate the effects of fatigue among medical personnel on rates of medical errors or adverse events would be useful. In the meantime, the lack of convincing data linking fatigue with poor patient outcomes should not deter us from tackling the issue of fatigue among medical personnel.

Practice Descriptions

Hours of Service

We reviewed the evidence for 2 potential safety practices concerning hours of service: 8-hour versus 12-hour length shifts and regulations limiting maximum shift length and/ or total hours worked. Most observational studies on optimal shift length to reduce fatigue and maximise performance are in non-medical settings and present inconsistent findings. In a study of work-place accidents in Germany, Hanecke et al found accident risk increased exponentially after the 9 hour at work and was highest among workers whose shift began in the evening or night. The authors concluded that shifts that last longer than 8 hours might lead to more worker fatigue and higher risk of accidents. Axelsson and colleagues studied workers at a power plant and found no difference in sleepiness or performance between those who worked 8-hour shifts and those who worked 12-hour shifts. Another group found that switching from 8- to 12-hour shifts led to increased alertness on the job and improved recovery time after night shifts. Overland has proposed that work that requires complex cognitive tasks may be ill suited for longer shifts, whereas work with limited cognitive demands may be well suited for longer shifts. Because the components of work vary dramatically within and across industries, shift durations that maintain performance in one setting may be ineffective in another.

We identified 9 observational studies comparing 8- versus 12-hour shifts for medical personnel. Two studies of nursing care on 10 wards found that quantity and quality of care were significantly lower with 12-hour shifts. Six studies of nurses and one of physicians measured outcomes including self-reported alertness, self-reported performance, and/or worker satisfaction. While 2 nurse studies found that self-reported alertness, performance, and satisfaction wane with longer shifts, Urgovics and Wright found that ICU nurses reported higher job satisfaction and subjectively improved clinical performance with 12-hour shifts. The 3 remaining studies in nurses found no difference in either satisfaction or self-reported performance between 8- and 12-hour shifts. A survey of emergency department physicians found that those who worked 12-hour shifts were less likely to be satisfied than those who worked 8-hour shifts. The relationship between these subjective outcomes measures and medical error is not clear.

Hours of service regulations as an effort to reduce errors due to fatigue are standard in some non-medical fields. Truck drivers are typically allowed to work no more than 10 hours at a time and no more than 60 hours in one week. Airline pilots and air traffic controllers work regulated hours and some data suggest waning performance as work-hours increase. Although most healthcare personnel are not subject to work-hour standards, many physicians-in-training are, either by statutory regulations or by being in an accredited training programme. In a retrospective cohort study, Laine and colleagues found the aforementioned New York State regulations limiting resident work-hours had no effect on patient outcomes such as mortality or transfers to the intensive care unit but were associated with increased rates of medical complications and delays in diagnostic tests. These negative effects may have been related to discontinuity of care and/or fewer physician-hours per patient. As the authors noted, "better care may be provided by a tired physician who is familiar with the patient than by a rested physician who is less familiar with the patient." In a case-control study, Petersen and colleagues found that when patients were cared for by a physician other than their primary resident, they were 6 times as likely to suffer a preventable adverse event. Thus, fewer physician work hours may lead to more physician discontinuity and potentially, more adverse events and poorer outcomes for patients. On the other hand, Gottlieb studied changes in a medical service staffing schedule that allowed for reduced sleep deprivation, improved distribution of admissions throughout the week, and improved continuity of inpatient care. After these changes were instituted, patients had shorter lengths of stay, fewer ancillary tests, and fewer medication errors.

Although it is difficult to ascribe the improvements to changes in work-hours because several other changes were made as well, it does appear that changes in work-hours can be made without adversely affecting patient outcomes. Any effort to change duty hours for healthcare personnel in an effort to reduce fatigue should factor in and continuously monitor numerous variables, including the potential costs of discontinuity, medical complications and unnecessary hospital days, to ensure that the measures do not compromise patient care. The costs needed to maintain adequate staffing in face of lost physician work-hours has been estimated to be $360 million in New York State alone. However, the difficult task of estimating other costs and potential savings from implementing these regulations has not been accomplished. Finally, some authors have expressed concern that restriction of resident physician work-hours may lead to poorer quality training and decreased professionalism among doctors. They argue that restricted working hours will decrease a sense of obligation to patients and will sanction self-interest over the well-being of patients. However, there are no data to substantiate these concerns.

Improving Sleep: Education about Sleep Hygiene

Good sleep hygiene, including the avoidance of alcohol and caffeine before bedtime, and maintaining a healthy sleep environment, may aid in decreasing sleep debt and fatigue. Studies of sleep hygiene have focused on treatment of persons with insomnia or other chronic sleep disorders. We found no clinical studies that measure the efficacy of good sleep hygiene among shift workers. Generally, most employers cannot dictate how their workers spend their hours off-duty and compliance with recommendations may be poor. One study of law-enforcement officers working rotating shifts found significant increases in awareness and knowledge after a training session on sleep hygiene practices but no change on a post-sleep inventory assessed at one-month follow-up. The effectiveness of educational programmes about sleep hygiene to improve shift worker performance requires further study.

Lighting at Work

The body's regulation of circadian rhythm is mediated by the effects of light and darkness. A 1986 survey found that 7.3 million Americans work at night. These employees, who work during dark hours and sleep during daylight hours, are often chronically sleep deprived and may suffer adverse health effects, partially due to poor synchrony of circadian rhythm to work schedule. Since scheduled light exposure can produce a phase shift in the endogenous circadian rhythm, investigators have studied changes in lighting at work and home to improve adjustment to the shift cycle. Foret et al studied 8 young men in a sleep lab and found exposure to bright lights during the night produced a beneficial effect on subjective alertness. Czeisler and colleagues found that subjects who were exposed to bright light at night and nearly complete darkness during the day had better cognitive performance and subjective alertness, and longer daytime sleep (7.7 vs. 5.7 hours, $p=0.01$). Manipulation of light and dark is much easier in sleep labs than in the field, where unintended exposure to bright light is common and may adversely impact attempts to alter workers' circadian rhythm.

The National Aeronautics and Space Administration (NASA) has studied the efficacy of bright lights on shuttle astronauts. Their encouraging results suggest that alterations in circadian rhythm can be obtained upon on exposure to light at night. The United States Nuclear Regulatory Commission has also implemented bright lighting for its night workers and found less fatigue and better alertness on the job. Field studies are needed to determine how bright artificial light affects objective measures of performance in healthcare workers and medical error. Bright light may not be appropriate for all areas of the hospital. For example, Bullough and Rea have noted that while bright light might help workers in neonatal care units, it may also be detrimental to patients. Nonetheless, lighting can be a relatively inexpensive intervention using existing equipment. Keeping lights bright at night, and educating workers about using heavy shades at home may have an important impact on worker performance on night shifts.

Medical Therapies

Melatonin is the major hormone responsible for circadian rhythm regulation. James et al studied the effect of oral melatonin supplementation on circadian rhythm and adaptation to night shifts among medical personnel. They and others have found no effect among medical shift workers. Though melatonin continues to be studied for chronic insomnia and other conditions, there currently is insufficient evidence to recommend its use to combat the fatigue associated with changing workshifts. Some studies have looked at the potential benefits of benzodiazepines and other sedatives for short-term insomnia associated with shift work, but no data exist on long-term use. Stimulants and caffeine can boost performance acutely but do not address the underlying sleep deprivation, and thus are not a viable long-term solution. Furthermore, concern over side effects, addiction, and performance degradation with current pharmacologic interventions makes their use as a safety practice unlikely.

Direction and Speed of Rotation of Shift Work

The direction of *shift rotation* may impact worker fatigue.

For workers who change from one shift to another, a forward rotation of shift work (morning shifts followed by evening shifts followed by night shifts) may lead to less fatigue on the job than backward rotation (day shift to night shift to evening shift). Forward rotation appears easier to tolerate physiologically since the natural circadian rhythm tends to move forward and it is more difficult to fall asleep earlier than the normal bedtime. Several studies in non-medical personnel have shown that forward rotation allows for better acclimation of the circadian rhythm. However, 2 other studies found no significant difference in forward versus backward shift rotation. None of these studies measured worker performance or error rates and we found no studies that evaluated direction of shift work rotation among medical personnel. Another variable in scheduling is the speed of shift work rotation. Studies suggest that slow rotation (e.g., changing from one shift to another every one to two weeks) may allow for better adaptation of the circadian rhythm than fast rotation (e.g., changing shifts every 2-3 days). Slow shift rotation results in greater sleep length at home, less sleepiness on the job, better self-reported performance, and fewer errors. In some cases, fast rotation may increase worker satisfaction but the effects of such satisfaction on safety have not been assessed. Shift rotation at an extremely slow rate approximates fixed, non-rotating shifts (permanent night shifts, permanent day shifts). Permanent shifts are associated with better adaptation to changes in the circadian rhythm and better performance than rotating shifts. However, daytime commitments and social obligations often prevent workers from completely adapting to permanent night shifts and worker satisfaction is poor.

Napping

Napping is common among shift workers and is perceived as a way to combat fatigue. One study of shift workers in a steel plant found that over half reported napping at home either before or after their shifts. The efficacy of naps has been studied in 3 settings: prior to periods of sleep deprivation (*prophylactic naps*), during periods of sleep deprivation (*therapeutic naps*) and during work hours (*maintenance naps*). Most studies have been conducted in sleep labs in healthy, young, male subjects. A number of studies in the non-medical literature have studied the efficacy of prophylactic napping. Gillberg and colleagues studied 8 male subjects who were allowed only 4 hours of sleep at night. When subjects took a 30-minute nap in the middle of the prior day, they had better subjective alertness, 20% improvement in vigilance performance, and less overall sleepiness than when they had not been allowed to nap. Others have also found benefits of prophylactic naps on subjective and objective measures of alertness and performance in healthy volunteers undergoing extended periods of sleep deprivation. Bonnet and Arand studied prophylactic versus therapeutic naps in 12 healthy young men who underwent 24 hours of sleep deprivation to simulate sleep patterns of medical housestaff. One group of subjects had a 4-hour prophylactic nap in the evening and caffeine during the 24 hours, while the second group had four, 1-hour naps during the 24-hour work period and no caffeine. Those in the prophylactic nap and caffeine group had a 15% increase in reasoning and overall improved subjective alertness compared with the group that had only short naps. There was no impact on mood. We identified one study of napping by medical personnel. Harma and colleagues studied 146 female hospital nurses and nurses' aides and found that those who napped prior to their night shifts were less likely to report on the job fatigue.

Most studies evaluating the efficacy of therapeutic napping during prolonged periods of sleep deprivation have found beneficial effects when compared with no napping. On the other hand, Gillberg and colleagues found no difference in simulated driving between the 2 groups of sleep deprived truck drivers, one group having taken a 30-minute nap during the middle of the previous night. Maintenance naps are naps that occur on the job, during the shift. These naps could compensate for daytime sleep deprivation or could bridge the nighttime low point in circadian somnolence. Many Japanese industries have provided their employees with the option of on the job napping and nearly half of nighttime shift workers take advantage of this opportunity. Though no systematic studies of the impact of maintenance naps exist in shift workers, one investigation found that short naps in the middle of the night improved performance for the rest of the shift. Napping over several successive shifts has not been studied. An important consideration in napping is the phenomena of *sleep inertia*, a period of transitory hypo-vigilance, confusion, disorientation of behaviour and impaired cognitive performance that immediately follows awakening. Sleep inertia is well documented and lasts up to 30 minutes after awakening. The duration of deep sleep and the time of the nap, relative to the circadian cycle, seem most related to the severity of sleep inertia. Strategies for napping on the job to reduce fatigue should be designed to avoid possible detrimental effects of sleep inertia.

Another potential negative effect of lengthy naps is that they can disrupt the quantity and quality of later sleep periods. In summary, there is strong evidence that therapeutic naps and maintenance naps combat the effects of fatigue and sleep loss. They can help subjects adapt better to circadian rhythm disturbances and perform better during acute sleep deprivation. Their application in the medical field is not well known. While prophylactic and therapeutic napping result in loss of social time at home, maintenance napping results in loss of work time. Costs associated with naps have not been reported. The financial impact of reduced worker fatigue due to napping has not been evaluated in medicine.

Comment

Sleep deprivation and disturbances of circadian rhythm lead to fatigue, decreased alertness, and poor performance on standardized testing. Although data from non-medical fields suggest that sleep deprivation leads to poor job performance, this link has not yet been established in medicine. Although the link with fatigue seems intuitive, promoting interventions designed to combat medical errors should be evidence-based. Limits on physician duty hours must account for potentially detrimental effects of discontinuity in patient care. Forward rather than backward shift rotation, education about good sleep hygiene, and strategic napping before or during shifts may reduce fatigue and improve performance. High face validity, low likelihood of harm, and ease of implementation make these promising strategies, although more evidence of their effectiveness in medicine is warranted. Studies on the use of bright light in the medical workplace are needed before it can be embraced. As Gaba points out, in most high-hazard industries the assumption is that fatigue and long, aberrant work hours lead to poor performance, and the burden of proof is in the hands of those who believe that such work practices are safe.

In medicine, concerns over discontinuity of care, and difficulties in changing medical culture have pushed the burden of proof into the hands of those who wish to change the *status quo*. Given that medical personnel, like all human beings, probably function suboptimally when fatigued, efforts to reduce fatigue and sleepiness should be undertaken, and the burden of proof should be in the hands of the advocates of the current system to demonstrate that it is safe. Finally, fatigue among medical personnel may not be fully remediable and human errors are, in the end, inevitable. The ultimate solution for healthcare organisations will likely require a systems-based approach that both limits the potential for human error and intercepts errors that do occur before they reach patients.

REFERENCES

Bailey KR. Generalizing the results of randomized clinical trials. *Control Clin Trials* 1994; 15:15-23.

Bates DW, Boyle DL, Vander Vliet MB, Schneider J, Leape L. Relationship between medication errors and adverse drug events. *J Gen Intern Med* 1995; 10:199-205.

Bates DW, Cullen DJ, Laird N, Petersen LA, Small SD, Servi D, et al. Incidence of adverse drug events and potential adverse drug events: Implications for prevention. *JAMA* 1995; 274:29-34.

Concato J, Shah N, Horwitz RI. Randomized, controlled trials, observational studies, and the hierarchy of research designs. *N Engl J Med* 2000; 342:1887-1892.

Cook DJ, Guyatt GH, Laupacis A, Sackett DL, Goldberg RJ. Clinical recommendations using levels of evidence for antithrombotic agents. *Chest* 1995; 108:227S-230S.

Cullen DJ, Sweitzer BJ, Bates DW, Burdick E, Edmondson A, Leape LL. Preventable adverse drug events in hospitalized patients: a comparative study of intensive care and general care units. *Crit Care Med* 1997; 25:1289-1297.

Felkey BG, Barker KN. Technology and automation in pharmaceutical care. *J Am Pharm Assoc (Wash)* 1996; NS36:309-314.

Glanville J, Lefebvre C. Identifying systematic reviews: key resources. *ACP J Club* 2000; 132:A11-A12.

Gotzsche PC, Liberati A, Torri V, Rossetti L. Beware of surrogate outcome measures. *Int J Technol Assess Health Care* 1996; 12:238-246.

Guerrero RM, Nickman NA, Jorgenson JA. Work activities before and after implementation of an automated dispensing system. *Am J Health Syst Pharm* 1996; 53:548-554.

Guyatt G, Schunemann H, Cook D, Jaeschke R, Pauker S, Bucher H. Grades of recommendation for antithrombotic agents. *Chest* 2001; 119:3S-7S.

Guyatt GH, Sackett DL, Sinclair JC, Hayward R, Cook DJ, Cook RJ. Users' guides to the medical literature. IX. A method for grading health care recommendations. Evidence-Based Medicine Working Group. *JAMA* 1995; 274:1800-1804.

Guyatt GH, Tugwell PX, Feeny DH, Drummond MF, Haynes RB. The role of before-after studies of therapeutic impact in the evaluation of diagnostic technologies. *J Chronic Dis* 1986; 39:295-304.

Harris RP, Helfand M, Woolf SH, Lohr KN, Mulrow CD, Teutsch SM, et al. Current methods of the U.S. Preventive Services Task Force. A review of the process. *Am J Prev Med* 2001; 20:21-35.

Hunt DL, McKibbon KA. Locating and appraising systematic reviews. *Ann Intern Med* 1997; 126:532-538.

Jadad AR, Cook DJ, Browman GP. A guide to interpreting discordant systematic reviews. *CMAJ* 1997; 156:1411-1416.

Juni P, Witschi A, Bloch R, Egger M. The hazards of scoring the quality of clinical trials for meta-analysis. *JAMA* 1999; 282:1054-1060.

Klein EG, Santora JA, Pascale PM, Kitrenos JG. Medication cart-filling time, accuracy, and cost with an automated dispensing system. *Am J Hosp Pharm* 1994; 51:1193-1196.

Levine M, Walter S, Lee H, Haines T, Holbrook A, Moyer V. Users' guides to the medical literature. IV. How to use an article about harm. Evidence-Based Medicine Working Group. *JAMA* 1994; 271:1615-1619.

McAuley L, Pham B, Tugwell P, Moher D. Does the inclusion of grey literature influence estimates of intervention effectiveness reported in meta-analyses? *Lancet* 2000; 356:1228-1231.

McKee M, Britton A, Black N, McPherson K, Sanderson C, Bain C. Methods in health services research. Interpreting the evidence: choosing between randomised and non-randomised studies. *BMJ* 1999; 319:312-315.

Mulrow C, Langhorne P, Grimshaw J. Integrating heterogeneous pieces of evidence in systematic reviews. *Ann Intern Med* 1997; 127:989-995.

Perini VJ, Vermeulen LC, Jr. Comparison of automated medication-management systems. *Am J Hosp Pharm* 1994; 51:1883-1891.

Ringold DJ, Santell JP, Schneider PJ. ASHP national survey of pharmacy practice in acute care settings: dispensing and administration—1999. *Am J Health Syst Pharm* 2000; 57:1759-1775.

Schwarz HO, Brodowy BA. Implementation and evaluation of an automated dispensing system. *Am J Health Syst Pharm* 1995; 52:823-828.

Shirley KL. Effect of an automated dispensing system on medication administration time. *Am J Health Syst Pharm* 1999; 56:1542-1545.

2

Medical Faculty Organisation

History of the School

The School of Medicine traces its origin to the first medical school on the Pacific Coast, founded in San Francisco by Dr. Elias Samuel Cooper as the Medical Department of the University of the Pacific in 1858. Stanford University was founded in 1885. In 1908, the University's Board of Trustees adopted Cooper Medical College as the University's School of Medicine. The School moved from San Francisco to the Stanford University campus in 1959.

Mission of the School of Medicine

The Stanford University School of Medicine provides an educational environment that encourages intellectual diversity and offers stimulation and opportunity for self-motivated students who are interested in developing a scholarly, investigative approach to problems in medicine.

The Mission Statement for the MD Degree Programme of the Stanford University School of Medicine, approved by the Senate of the School of Medicine Faculty Council on June 14, 2000 is:

— To educate future physicians and foster their capacity to make discoveries and lead innovation in the science and practice of medicine

The Educational Goals for the MD Degree Programme, Stanford University School of Medicine, revised and approved by the Senate of the School of Medicine Faculty Council, June 14, 2000 are:

1. To assure excellence in clinical medicine with emphasis on:
   a. Understanding the traditional and emerging areas of biomedical and clinical sciences, including the etiology, prevention, diagnosis and treatment of disease
   b. Understanding the scientific theory and methodology that form the basis of medical discoveries
   c. Utilizing opportunities to explore research and teaching, both broadly defined, in various branches of medicine, with access to the full resources of Stanford University
   d. Using technology to manage information and knowledge effectively and efficiently
2. To develop effective communication skills with patients, colleagues and the public
3. To promote leadership training in the various branches of medicine
4. To promote ethical and moral behavior, the humane and caring practice of medicine and a sense of obligation to improve the health of the public
5. To promote cultural competency in the science and practice of medicine
6. To teach the skills necessary to sustain a lifetime of learning

The admissions process is directed to the selection of

individuals who will most benefit from this environment. Recognizing the importance of a diverse student body providing a rich educational experience, the School has a strong commitment to identify, recruit and educate students from a wide variety of backgrounds, including minority groups and women.

School of Medicine Vision for the Twenty-First Century

Our school is one of the nation's preeminent institutions for education, biomedical research and clinical care. This will not change. In our vision for the 21st century, we shall continue to be recognized for our extraordinary ability to make fundamental discoveries in biology and biomedical sciences. But we shall also be focused on translating those discoveries into diagnostic and therapeutic applications for improved patient care. We shall institute policies and structures that will encourage productive collaborations, and facilitate the movement from fundamental discoveries to diagnosis and treatment of disease. We shall continue to attract and retain the highest quality faculty members who will work collectively and who will have the experience, knowledge and insight necessary to respond to new research and programmatic opportunities and to be a central focus for excellence in patient care. We shall continue to create unparalleled educational opportunities for our medical students, graduate students, fellows and house staff physicians, and to prepare them for leadership careers in medicine and biomedical research.

Our medical students will leave intellectually prepared both to grasp and contribute to the growing body of biomedical knowledge and emotionally prepared to care for patients with compassion and respect. Our graduate students and fellows will conduct important basic and clinical research with extraordinary faculty and will leave prepared for career both within and outside academia. Our medical school community will reflect the richness of America's communities and will foster a supportive, hospitable environment that encourages the fullest extent of intellectual and personal development for all. Finally, we shall continue to benefit from being part of a world class university and will take advantage of the opportunities of integration–those that arise from the interface between medicine and other disciplines, from a sharing of ideas, resources and technology, and from access to the rich intellectual environment of the University as a whole.

School of Medicine Deans

John Maxson Stillman—*Acting Executive Head 1910,1911*

Ray Lyman Wilbur (1875,1949)—*Dean 1911,1916*

William Ophuls (1871,1933)—*Dean 1916-1933*

Loren Roscoe Chandler (1895,1982)—*Dean 1933-1953*

Windsor C. Cutting (1907,1972)—*Dean 1953-1957*

Robert H. Alway—*Acting Dean 1957,1958—Dean 1958,1964*

Sidney Raffel—*Acting Dean 1964,1965*

Robert J. Glaser—*Dean 1965,1970*

John Wilson—*Acting Dean 1970,1971*

Clayton Rich—*Dean 1971,1978*

Lawrence G. Crowley—*Acting Dean 1979,1981*

Dominick P. Purpura—*Dean 1982,1984*

David Korn—*Dean 1984,1995*

Eugene A. Bauer, MD—*Dean 1995,2001*

Philip A. Pizzo, MD—*Dean 2001*

History of the School of Medicine

1851 University of the Pacific, oldest chartered college in California, founded in Santa Clara.

1858 Dr. Elias Samuel Cooper (1822—1862) founds University of the Pacific Medical Department in San Francisco.

1861 Dr. Levi Cooper Lane (d. 1902), Cooper's nephew, joins faculty.

1864 Medical Department operations suspended because some faculty, including Lane, moved to Toland Medical College–later to become University of California School of Medicine–which opened in San Francisco.

1870 Lane and close associates resigned Toland, reorganized Medical Department of University of the Pacific with Henry Gibbons Jr., MD (1840—1911), who had received his MD from the Department in 1863, as Dean.

1872 Medical Department became known as Medical College of the Pacific when, in order to gain access to better classroom facilities, the faculty amicably arranged to have it transferred to University (City) College.

1882 Lane donated new building at Sacramento and Webster Streets. Name changed to Cooper Medical College. Said to be the best facility for medical education in the world, that building was in continuous use until 1959.

1890 Lane donated addition that doubled size of medical school, included lecture halls, labs and other facilities.

1893-4 Lane donated and raised funds for construction of Lane Hospital at Clay and Webster Streets.

1895 Lane Hospital Training School for Nurses (later Stanford School of Nursing) established. Lane Hospital inaugurated.

1908 Board of Directors of Cooper Medical College grants its San Francisco properties and equipment to Stanford University. The College becomes the Medical Department of Stanford University. Clinical programmes and some basic science courses continue at San Francisco facilities; some basic sciences taught on campus.

1901 First class admitted to Stanford University School of Medicine.

1912 Last class graduates Cooper. Lane Medical Library, finest collection west of Chicago, moves to new building, financed by an advance from Stanford and a gift from Cooper Medical College, at Webster and Sacramento.

1917 Stanford Hospital opens on Clay Street, adjoining Lane Hospital, to provide additional beds and clinical teaching facilities. The two are known as Stanford Lane Hospital.

1953 Stanford's Board of Trustees makes decision to move Medical School from San Francisco to Campus.

1959 The School of Medicine, Clinics and Palo Alto-Stanford Hospital become Stanford University Medical Center; opens on campus. Palo Alto-Stanford Hospital was financed jointly by the University and the city of Palo Alto to secure teaching, research and clinical resources for the University and hospital beds for Palo Alto patients.

1968 Stanford purchased Palo Alto's entire interest and renamed the hospital Stanford University Hospital.

1994 The Faculty Practice merged with Stanford University Hospital to form Stanford Health Services.

1997 Lucile Packard Children's Hospital merged with Stanford Health Services. Stanford Health Services merged with University of California San Francisco Medical Center and UCSF Faculty Practice in the first such merger of its kind between private and state medical centers, known as UCSF Stanford Health Care.

1999 UCSF Stanford Health Care merger dissolved to form Stanford Hospital and Clinics and Lucile Packard Children's Hospital.

Medical Faculty Organization

Administrative Structure of the School of Medicine

Dean

Appointment to this position is made by the President of the University after consultation with the Advisory Board and is reported to the Board of Trustees. The Dean serves at the will of the President. The Dean may also serve, at the will of the President, as Vice President for the Medical Center. On matters relating to Medical Center governance, the Dean reports to the Vice President for the Medical Center. On academic matters concerning the School, the Dean reports to the Provost

Associate Deans

The establishment of a new position of Associate Dean is recommended by the Dean and approved by the Provost. Appointment to the position of Associate Dean is recommended to the Provost by the Dean after consultation with the Executive Committee of the School. After the Provost approves the appointment, the President reports it to the Board of Trustees. An Associate Dean serves at the will of the Dean.

Senior Associate Deans

The establishment of a new position of Senior Associate Dean is recommended by the Dean and approved by the Provost. Appointment to the position of Senior Associate Dean is recommended to the Provost by the Dean after consultation with the Executive Committee of the School. After the Provost approves the appointment, the President reports it to the Board of Trustees. A Senior Associate Dean serves at the will of the Dean.

Assistant Deans

The establishment of a new position of Assistant Dean is recommended by the Dean and approved by the Provost. Appointment to the position of Assistant Dean is recommended by the Dean and approved by the Provost. An Assistant Dean serves at the will of the Dean.

The Medical Center

Stanford University Medical Center consists of the School of Medicine, Stanford Hospital and Clinics and Lucile Salter Packard Children¼s Hospital.

Chief Executive Officer of Stanford Hospital and Clinics

Appointment to this position is nominated by the Vice President and approved by the Board of Directors of Stanford Hospital and Clinics. The Chief Executive Officer of Stanford Hospital and Clinics reports to the Vice President and the Board of Directors and is a member of the Boards of Directors of both Stanford Hospital and Clinics and Lucile Salter Packard Children¼s Hospital. The Chief Executive Officer is subject to removal by the Board of Directors of Stanford Hospital and Clinics.

Chief Executive Officer of Lucile Salter Packard Children¼s Hospital

Appointment to this position is nominated by the Vice President and approved by the Board of Directors of Lucile Salter Packard Children's Hospital. The Chief Executive Officer of Lucile Salter Packard Children's Hospital reports to the Vice President and the Board of Directors and is a member of the Boards of Directors of both Stanford Hospital and Clinics and Lucile Salter Packard Children¼s Hospital. The Chief Executive Officer is subject to removal by the Board of Directors of Lucile Salter Packard Children's Hospital.

Vice President for the Medical Center

Appointment to this position is made by the President of the University after consultation with the Advisory Board and is reported to the Board of Trustees. The Vice President for the Medical Center is a member of the Boards of Directors of both Stanford Hospital and Clinics and Lucile Salter Packard Children¼s Hospital. The Vice President for the Medical Center reports to and serves at the will of the President of the University.

Departmental Structure

The establishment or abolition of an academic department is recommended by the Dean to the Provost after consulting the Executive Committee of the School. If the Provost recommends approval, the proposal is forwarded to the Advisory Board, which submits a recommendation to the President. The President, in turn, recommends it to the Board of Trustees, which makes the final decision. The rationale for giving departmental status to an academic activity must be strong and well supported by documentation of programmatic need and meeting financial and other requirements. There are currently twenty-six academic departments within the School of Medicine.

Clinical Sciences Departments

1. Anesthesia
2. Cardiothoracic Surgery
3. Comparative Medicine
4. Dermatology

5. Functional Restoration
6. Gynecology & Obstetrics
7. Medicine
8. Neurology & Neurological Sciences
9. Neurosurgery
10. Ophthalmology
11. Otolaryngology
12. Pathology
13. Pediatrics
14. Psychiatry & Behavioral Sciences
15. Radiation Oncology
16. Radiology
17. Surgery
18. Urology

Basic Sciences Departments

1. Biochemistry
2. Bioengineering
3. Developmental Biology
4. Genetics
5. Health Research & Policy
6. Microbiology & Immunology
7. Molecular and Cellular Physiology
8. Molecular Pharmacology
9. Neurobiology
10. Structural Biology

Department Chairs

A candidate for chair of a department is identified by

search or other procedure decided by the Dean, who recommends appointment to the Provost after consultation with the Executive Committee of the School. The Provost, acting on behalf of the President and after appropriate consultation, approves the appointment. The President reports it to the Board of Trustees. The department chair serves at the will of the President and the Dean. The chair, as administrative head of the department, is responsible to the Dean in matters concerning the departmental operating budget, personnel actions and similar matters.

Acting Department Chairs

An acting chair is appointed to perform the duties of a chair on a temporary basis. The procedure for appointment and termination of an acting chair is the same as for the appointment of a chair.

Associate Chairs of Departments

An associate chair is appointed by the Dean on the recommendation of the chair who states the reasons for the recommendation and the qualifications of the candidate for the assignment. The associate chair serves at the will of the Dean, contingent upon the continued support of the chair.

Departmental Divisions

A departmental division may be established by the Dean on recommendation of the department chair, who states the academic and administrative reasons and documents the personnel, fiscal, space and other requirements. Divisional status is reserved for academic activities sufficiently distinctive, extensive and significant to require administrative differentiation for optimum development and management.

Division Chiefs

The chief of a division is appointed by the Dean on recommendation of the department chair, and serves at the will of the Dean contingent upon the continued support of the chair.

Executive Committee

The Executive Committee of the School is composed of the following voting members: the Dean (chair of the committee), the chairs of the academic departments of the School, a representative of the Interdepartmental Programmes, and the representative of the Faculty Council. Nonvoting members are designated by the Dean and currently include the Senior Associate Deans and the Associate Dean for Academic Affairs. The committee is a major consultative body of the School and is advisory to the Dean, who determines the agenda. The Executive Committee considers confidential matters such as appointments, reappointments and promotions and may consider, at the request of the Dean, and all policies of the School.

School of Medicine Executive Organization

President—John L. Hennessy

Provost—John W. Etchemendy

Vice President for the Medical Center—Eugene A. Bauer, MD

Associate Vice President for Medical Development & Alumni Affairs—Jacquelyn Brown

Dean—Philip A. Pizzo, MD

Senior Associate Dean for Academic Affairs—David Stevenson, MD

Senior Associate Dean for Clinical Affairs—Peter B. Gregory, MD

Senior Associate Dean for Education & Student Affairs—Pending

Senior Associate Dean for Finance & Administration—Michael A. Hindery

Senior Associate Dean for Research—W. James Nelson, PhD

Associate Dean for Alumni Affairs—Ross Bright, MD

Associate Dean for Veteran's Affairs—Javaid Sheikh, MD

Associate Dean for Student Services—Michael Cowan

Associate Dean for Preclinical Advising & Research—Patricia Cross, PhD

Associate Dean for Continuing Education—Bertil Glader, MD

Associate Dean for Minority Advising & Programmes—Fernando Mendoza, MD

Associate Dean for Graduate Affairs—Ellen Porzig, PhD

Associate Dean for Clinical Advising & Professional Transition—Elliott Wolfe, MD

Associate Dean for Education & Graduate Affairs—Neil Gesundheit, MD

Assistant Dean for Academic Affairs—Linda Deasy

Assistant Dean for Minority Affairs—Ronald Garcia, PhD

Chairs of Clinical Sciences

Anesthesia —Ronald G. Pearl, MD, PhD

Cardiothoracic Surgery—Bruce A. Reitz, MD

Comparative Medicine—Linda C. Cork, DVM, PhD

Dermatology—Alfred T. Lane, MD

Functional Restoration—Stephen A. Schendel. MD, DDS

Gynecology & Obstetrics—Mary Lake Polan, MD, PhD

Medicine—Judith L. Swain, MD

Neurology & Neurological Sciences—William C. Mobley, MD, PhD

Neurosurgery—Gary K. Steinberg, MD, PhD

Ophthalmology—Mark S. Blumenkranz, MD

Pathology—Stephen J. Galli, MD

Pediatrics—Harvey J. Cohen, MD, PhD

Psychiatry & Behavioral Sciences—Alan F. Schatzberg, MD

Radiology—Gary M. Glazer, MD

Radiation Oncology—Richard T. Hoppe, MD

Surgery—Thomas M. Krummel, MD

Urology—Linda Shortliffe, MD

Chairs of Basic Sciences

Biochemistry—Suzanne Pfeffer, PhD

Developmental Biology—Roeland Nusse, PhD

Genetics—David Botstein, PhD

Health Research & Policy—Mark A. Hlatky, MD

Microbiology & Immunology—John C. Boothroyd, PhD

Molecular & Cellular Physiology—W. James Nelson, PhD

Molecular Pharmacology—Helen M. Blau, PhD

Neurobiology—Eric Knudsen, PhD

Structural Biology—Michael Levitt, PhD

Faculty

The faculty of the School of Medicine consists of the Academic Council Professoriate and the Medical Center Line.

Academic Council Professoriate

The Academic Council Professoriate includes Tenure Line faculty at all ranks and Non-Tenure Line faculty at all ranks. The latter consists of three lines: the Clinical Line (to which there have been no new appointments since 1989), the Research Line and the Teaching Line. For definitions and additional information concerning University Governance.

Staff

Academic Staff

Teaching Staff, which includes Lecturers and Senior Lecturers, are appointed by the Senior Associate Dean for Academic Affairs upon recommendation from the Department Chair.

Research Staff, which includes Research Associate, Senior Research Scientist or Scholar, and Senior Research Engineer, are appointed upon recommendation from the Department Chair.

University Staff

Staff Physicians are appointed by the Senior Associate Dean for Academic Affairs upon the recommendation of the Department Chair. Because an appointment to the University Staff as Staff Physician involves teaching, a coterminous appointment to the Voluntary Clinical Faculty is required.

Other Teaching Titles

Other titles include Professor Emeritus (Active) and Assistant, Associate or full Professor (by courtesy), which are faculty titles. Acting Faculty, Visiting Faculty, Consulting Faculty, and Voluntary Clinical Faculty are teaching titles, but are not members of the School of Medicine faculty.

The Faculty Council of the School of Medicine

The Faculty Council of the School includes all faculty members in the School who hold primary or joint appointments in the School.

The Senate of the Faculty Council of the School of Medicine (Faculty Council Senate)

The Faculty Council Senate of the School is composed of Departmental Senators (one from each Department), two Senators-at-Large (one from the Clinical Science Departments and one from the Basic Science Departments) and one faculty representative of the interdisciplinary programmes and centers, all of whom are elected by the members of the Faculty Council in their respective units; and the Dean of the School, who is an ex officio member.

The purpose of the Senate is to represent the will and opinion of the School faculty in the deliberation and decision-making processes of the School, in formulating the curriculum for its students, and in promoting communication among its faculty, students and administrative officers. A Committee of Five, composed of two representatives from the Basic Sciences departments, two from the Clinical Sciences departments and a chair from either group, functions as the executive committee of the Senate. Responsibility for all aspects of medical student education is vested in the Senate through its four standing committees:

— Committee on Admissions (CA) is responsible for all aspects of the identification and selection process for the medical student entering class.

— Committee on Courses and Curriculum (CCC)

oversees all aspects of the medical student curriculum

- Committee on Student Performance (CSP) reviews the academic progress and problems of students and prescribes academic programmes to assist the students in correcting deficiencies and achieving the goal of acquiring the MD degree.
- Medical Student Scholars Committee (MSSC) is responsible for reviewing medical student research proposals, determining research awards and establishing criteria for project completion.

The powers and functions of the Faculty Council Senate of the School and its standing committees are detailed in the *Articles of Organization for the Senate of the Stanford University School of Medicine Faculty Council* below.

Articles of Organization for the Senate of the Stanford University School of Medicine Faculty Council (Amended August 1999)

The faculty of the Stanford University School of Medicine in order to participate fully in the deliberation and decision-making processes of this School, formulate the curriculum for its students, and promote the communication between its faculty, students and administrative officers, does establish a Senate according to these Articles of Organization, and subject to the provisions of the Articles of Organization of the Faculty of Stanford University.

Article I: The Powers & Functions of the Senate

Section 1

The Senate shall represent the will and the opinion of the faculty of the School.

Section 2

For the degree of Doctor of Medicine, the Senate shall

have the power to determine the requirements for admission of candidates; to define the curriculum; to establish criteria for student standing and promotion; and to determine the administration of the Medical Student Scholar research fellowships. The Senate shall be concerned with the establishment of policy on these matters and in so doing shall seek the advice of the Dean and the Executive Committee. The implementation of these policies shall be the function of the Dean and the Executive Committee.

For the degree of Doctor of Philosophy and Master of Science, the Senate shall act in an advisory capacity on matters concerning admission of candidates, curriculum, and student standing and promotion. In so doing, the Senate will confer with representatives of the graduate programmes, members of the Executive Committee, and the Dean.

The Senate shall advise on academic matters of house staff in Stanford Hospital and its affiliated hospitals.

The Senate shall advise on academic matters of postdoctoral students in the School of Medicine.

The Senate shall advise School of Medicine faculty on matters of faculty welfare and legal representation.

Section 3

The Senate shall give its advice on any other matters it deems relevant to the general welfare of the School, its faculty, its medical students, graduate students, postdoctoral students, and its house staff.

Article II: The Composition & Election of the Senate

Section 1

The Senate shall be composed of Departmental Senators and Senators-at-Large, elected by the members of the electorate in the respective electoral units, one faculty representative of the Interdisciplinary Programmes and Centers (IDPs), and the Dean of the School who shall be an ex-officio member of the Senate. Each Senator, including the Dean and the IDP representative, shall have one vote.

Section 2

Members of the electorate shall consist of all members of the Faculty Council of the School of Medicine who hold an appointment other than by courtesy in the Medical School. The Faculty Council includes faculty members who are members of the Academic Council of the University and those who are appointed in the Medical Center Line.

Section 3

Two types of electoral unit shall exist, "Departmental" and "At Large." A Departmental Unit shall consist of the members of the electorate in a department. The two "At Large" units shall be termed the BMS unit and the Clinical Unit. The BMS Unit shall consist of members of the electorate in the BMS departments and the Clinical Unit shall consist of the members of the electorate in the clinical departments. Members of the electorate who are not affiliated with departments shall vote in either the Clinical or BMS Unit as determined by the Chairperson of the Senate. The BMS departments are Biochemistry, Developmental Biology, Genetics, Health Research and Policy, Microbiology and Immunology, Molecular and Cellular Physiology, Molecular Pharmacology, Neurobiology, Pathology, and Structural Biology. The clinical departments are Anesthesia, Cardiothoracic Surgery, Comparative Medicine, Dermatology, Functional Restoration, Gynecology and Obstetrics, Medicine, Neurology and Neurological Sciences, Neurosurgery, Ophthalmology, Pediatrics, Psychiatry and Behavioral Sciences, Radiation Oncology, Radiology, Surgery, Urology.

Section 4

(1) The Departmental Senators shall be elected for a term of three years by, and from among, the members of the electorate in the respective Departmental Units, the number of Senators to be determined by the number of members in the Departmental Unit. Departmental Units containing one to twenty members shall elect one Senator; Departmental Units containing twenty-one to forty members shall elect two Senators; and Departmental Units containing more than forty members shall elect three Senators. Each Departmental Unit shall elect a number of Alternates equal to the number of Senators it elects. The Alternates shall be ranked, so that a Second Alternate will be called upon only if the First Alternate is unavailable, and so on.

(2) The BMS and Clinical Senators-at-Large shall be elected for a term of three years by, and from among, the members of the electorate in the respective BMS and Clinical Units. The number of BMS Senators-at-Large shall equal the number of Clinical Senators-at-Large. The total number of Senators-at-Large shall be one-half the total number of Departmental Senators; if this result is not an even number, then the nearest larger even number shall equal the total number of Senators-at-Large. In the election of Senators-at-Large, three Alternates shall be designated in each of the two Units, and shall be ranked, according to the procedure described in the Standing Rules appended to these Articles of Organization. The Alternates shall be the persons highest on the preference list, and who are willing to serve, after the required number of Senators-at-Large has been elected.

(3) One voting faculty representative of the Interdisciplinary Programmes and Centers (IDPs) shall be selected according to a process agreed upon by the IDPs.

(4) Five nonvoting representatives in the Senate, with

the privilege of participation in debate, shall be selected as follows: A medical student, representing the medical students of the School, shall be chosen by a mechanism ratified by a majority of all medical students of the School. Similarly, a graduate student, representing the graduate students of the School, shall be chosen by a mechanism ratified by a majority of all graduate students of the School. A member of the Voluntary Clinical Faculty shall be either the duly-elected President of the Medical Staff of Stanford University Hospital or the duly-elected vice-president of the Medical Staff if the President is not a member of the Voluntary Clinical Faculty. If neither the President nor the vice-president of the Medical Staff is a member of the VCF, then a special election should be held by the Medical Staff according to their procedures. A representative of the Stanford Medical School Alumni Association shall be chosen by that organization. A house staff member representing the house staff of Stanford Hospital and its affiliated hospitals shall be chosen by a mechanism ratified by the majority of all the house staff members.

Section 5

Procedure for election of Departmental Senators and Senators-at-Large

(1) After January 31, the Committee of Five shall determine the number of Senators to be elected in each electoral unit according to Article II, Section 4, (1) and (2).

(2) Elections shall be held annually. The electoral process shall begin after February 15 and be completed for Senate membership by midsummer. Those elected shall begin their term the next September prior to the first regular meeting of the Senate held as specified in Article III, Section 3, (1).

(3) In all annual elections, Departmental Senators and Alternates shall be elected first, a majority of all those

voting being required for election. Each Department shall construct a list of the members of the electorate in its Department, excluding all Senators with one or two years yet to serve, members of the Department electorate who by leave of absence, sabbatical, or otherwise, shall be unable to perform the duties of Senator, and Senators completing their second consecutive three-year term. The members of the Departmental electorate shall vote by secret mail ballot for nominees, casting as many votes for Senators as the Department is entitled to by virtue of size. Calling the number to be elected from the Department N, then the 2N individuals receiving the largest number of votes shall become the nominees of that Department. The members of the Departmental electorate will then vote by secret mail ballot for N Senators from the list of nominees, and the N nominees receiving the highest preference will be elected. Departmental Units with 20 or less members may elect a one-stage procedure whereby the member receiving the highest number of votes in the election for nominees is selected as Senator.

(4) The Senators-at-Large shall then be elected as follows: A BMS and clinical list shall be constructed of the members of the electorate in the BMS and Clinical Units, excluding the newly-elected Departmental Senators, all Senators with one or two years yet to serve, members of the electorate in a Departmental Unit that already contributes two Senators-at-Large with one or two years yet to serve, members of the electorate who by leave of absence, Sabbatical, or otherwise, shall be unable to perform the duties of Senator, and Senators completing their second consecutive three-year term. The members of the electorate in the BMS Unit shall vote by secret mail ballot for nominees for Senators-at-Large and Alternates from the BMS list, each member casting as many votes as there are Senators-at-Large to be elected

from the BMS Unit, and the members of the electorate in the Clinical Unit shall vote in identical manner from the clinical list. Calling the number of Senators-at-Large to be elected from a given unit N, then the 2N + 3 individuals receiving the greatest number of votes in each Unit shall become the nominees of that Unit, with the proviso that there shall be no more than one nominee chosen from each Departmental Unit. The members of the electorate in a given Unit shall then vote by secret mail ballot for N Senators-at-Large and three alternate Senators-at-Large from among the 2N + 3 nominees in the Unit, ranking as many of the nominees as required, according to preference, as described in the Standing Rules, and the N + 3 individuals receiving the greatest preference in each Unit shall be elected as Senators and alternate Senators-at-Large.

(5) If a person who has been elected as a departmental Alternate is then elected Senator at Large, the department shall elect a replacement Alternate.

Section 6

(1) The maximum number of consecutive three year terms in the Senate to which any member of the electorate may be elected shall be two.

(2) Alternates elected or designated in the Departmental Unit or elected at Large serve for a one-year term. Department Chairs shall assign or elect alternate Senators equal in number to the number of departmental Senators and shall notify the Chair of the Senate by June 30 each year.

(3) Alternates in the same electoral unit shall be called upon, in order of their ranking, to serve in place of a Senator whenever that may be necessary by virtue of that Senator's inability to serve.

Article III: The Government of the Senate

Section 1

(1) The Chairperson shall have the responsibility of presiding over the meetings of the Senate, and the Committee of Five shall function as the executive committee of the Senate.

(2) The Chairperson (elected from either the BMS or Clinical unit), begins his or her Office the September prior to the first regular meeting of the Senate held as specified in Article III, Section 2,

(3). The Chairperson remains in office for one year and may be reelected as long as he or she continues to be a member of the Senate.

(4) The Committee of Five shall be composed of two representatives elected from the BMS unit and two representatives elected from the Clinical unit. Members of the Committee of Five serve two year staggered terms.

Section 2

Procedure for election of the Chair and members of the Committee of Five.

(1) Prior to the first meeting of the new Senate year, a Chairperson of the Senate and members of the Committee of Five shall be elected by mail ballot.

(2) A mail ballot shall be constructed containing the names of all Senators who have indicated willingness to serve as Chairperson of the Senate. The ballot shall be sent to all Senators, containing the names of all such Senators in alphabetical order, in order to select five nominees for the position of Chairperson of the Senate. A voter shall rank five names, and the five persons with the highest total preference scores shall be nominees. The Senate shall

elect a Chairperson from among the five nominees, employing a preference system of voting, as described in the Standing Rules.

(3) In the same manner, the entire Senate shall vote by mail ballot for members of the Committee of Five to fill the positions that are open in any given year. The Senators of the BMS Unit shall receive a mail ballot containing the names of all Senators in the BMS Unit, in alphabetical order, in order to select nominees for the BMS Unit positions on the Committee of Five. The Senators of the Clinical Unit shall, in like manner, vote to select nominees for the Clinical Unit positions on the Committee of Five. A ranking of the nominees of the BMS Unit and a separate ranking of those of the Clinical Unit will be distributed for preference voting. If the name of the newly elected Chairperson appears on either list of nominees, it shall be stricken. The BMS Unit Senators receiving the highest total preference score and the Clinical Unit Senators receiving the highest total preference score shall be declared elected to the Committee of Five.

(4) The Chairperson of the Senate of the preceding year, if not reelected to the Committee of Five, shall be a consultant member of that Committee, without vote, serving in addition to the elected members.

Section 3

(1) With the exception of the standing committees of the Senate described in Articles IV, V and VI, the Committee of Five shall appoint the members of all other committees created by the Senate.

(2) The Committee of Five shall have the option of appointing, in consultation with the Dean of the School, one member of the electorate to any committee created by

the Dean or Executive Committee of the School exclusive of this Executive Committee and the Appointments and Promotions Committee.

(3) The Chairperson of the Senate or a designate from among the members of the Committee of Five shall be a voting ex officio member of the Executive Committee of the School.

(4) If the Chairperson of the Senate is unable to serve out his or her one-year term, the Senate should elect a new Chairperson from the remaining four members of the Committee of Five according to the Standing Rules.

(5) The Committee of Five shall appoint an Executive Secretary of the Senate who shall serve for three years with one renewable term of three years. That appointment may be granted to a faculty member eligible for Senate membership or to a member of the staff deemed qualified to act in the role of Executive Secretary. Payment for this function shall come from a yearly discretionary budget negotiated with the Dean of the School of Medicine by the Committee of Five. The Executive Secretary serves as an ex-officio member of the Committee of Five. Duties of the Executive Secretary include assuring that Senate administration and business is conducted in accordance with the Articles of Organizations, preparing agendas in conjunction with the Chair, preparing Senate minutes and overseeing their distribution, assuring that the Senate archive is maintained, and other duties as directed by the Committee of Five.

Section 4

(1) The Committee of Five shall meet upon request of the Chairperson, and the presence of three of its voting members shall constitute a quorum for a meeting. Decisions shall be reached by majority vote of those present at a

meeting of the Committee of Five. The chairpersons of standing committees may be invited to attend meetings of the Committee of Five as ex-officio nonvoting members.

(2) The Committee of Five shall meet with the Dean at appropriate intervals for purposes of exchange of information.

(3) The Senate shall assemble for regular meetings each month from September through June. The Senate may decide at any meeting to omit the next regularly scheduled meeting except that of September. The Chairperson of the Senate may call special meetings of the Senate at any time. Special meetings may also be called by petition of twenty percent of the Senators to the Chairperson, by decision of the Committee of Five, or by request of the Dean of the School to the Chairperson. The Chairperson of the Senate shall call all special meetings within one week after the time specified in the request.

(4) Attendance by a majority of the membership of the Senate is expected at all meetings of the Senate. However, if attendance at any meeting does not meet the quorum requirements, then attendance by no less than 33% of the eligible voters will be sufficient to conduct business including official voting. Except as restricted elsewhere in these Articles, or by the Rules of Order, all actions of the Senate shall be by a majority of those in attendance.

(5) Agenda for regular meetings of the Senate shall be distributed to the electorate at least one week prior to the date of the meeting. The agenda for each regular meeting of the Senate shall provide opportunity for reports from the Dean and the Committee of Five. The student representatives, the representative of the voluntary clinical faculty, the alumni representative, the house staff representative, and the chairpersons of the standing committees may present reports to the Faculty Senate after submitting a request to

do so to the Committee of Five at least two weeks prior to the meeting date. Agenda for special meetings must be distributed prior to or at the time of the meeting.

(6) If the Chairperson is unable to preside over a scheduled meeting of the Senate, he or she should select a designate from the Committee of Five to chair the meeting.

(7) The Senate may determine the rules of its proceedings except as restricted in these Articles of Organization.

Article IV: Committees of Senate

Section 1

The major areas of Senate responsibility for matters pertaining to the degree of Doctor of Medicine–admissions, curriculum, student standing and promotion, administration of the Medical Student Scholars research fellowships–shall be dealt with by standing committees: a Committee on Medical Student Admissions (CA), a Committee on Medical Courses and Curriculum (CCC), a Committee on Medical Student Performance (CSP), a Medical Student Scholars Committee (MSSC).

Section 2

The three major areas of Senate responsibility for the degrees of Doctor of Philosophy and Master of Science–admissions, curriculum and student standing and promotion–shall be dealt with by three standing committees: a Committee on Graduate Admissions and Policy (CGAP), a Committee on Graduate Curriculum (CGC), and a Committee on Graduate Student Performance (CGSP).

Section 3

(1) Chairpersons of each of the standing committees shall be chosen by the Committee of Five, with the concurrence of the Dean, subject to confirmation by the

Senate. Except as otherwise specified in these Articles, members of the standing committees other than the chairpersons shall be recommended to the Committee of Five by the committee chairs, subject to confirmation by the Senate. All members of the standing committees, including the chairpersons, shall receive formal notice of appointment from the Dean and serve three year staggered terms that are renewable.

(2) Representation on CGAP and CGC shall also include representatives from each of the departmental and interdepartmental graduate programmes in the School of Medicine as well as faculty and student members from the graduate programmes in Biological Sciences and Biophysics.

(3) Medical students serving on CA or CCC shall be chosen yearly by a mechanism ratified by a majority of all medical students of the School. The names of the finalists will be submitted to the Office of Student Affairs for determination of eligibility, and the candidates confirmed by the Senate no later than its October meeting.

(4) Graduate students serving on CGAP or CGC shall be chosen yearly by a mechanism ratified by a majority of all graduate students in the Biosciences Programmes campus-wide. The names of the finalists will be submitted to the Office of Graduate Affairs for determination of eligibility, and the candidates confirmed by the Senate no later than its October meeting.

(5) Chairpersons and other members of standing committees except medical students and graduate students shall serve three-year staggered terms, renewable once, and shall then be eligible again for appointment only after an interval of three years.

(6) The Senate may, by two-thirds majority vote, remove

any or all members of a standing committee, including the chairperson.

(7) The Chairperson of each of the standing committee shall deliver to the Senate an annual report, which summarizes the activities of the committee during the preceding academic year.

Section 4

(1) The Senate may establish ad hoc committees for any purpose it deems desirable. The Committee of Five shall transmit to each ad hoc committee a written charge, representing the will of the Senate, and including a date by which a report is expected; and a copy of each such charge shall be communicated to the Senate and included in the Minutes of the Senate meetings that are sent to the electorate.

(2) Ad hoc committees, in general, shall consist of three to five members of the electorate appointed by the Committee of Five, but the Senate may, at its discretion, establish a larger committee in a given instance. When appropriate to the charge of an ad hoc committee, the Committee of Five may appoint to such committee a person other than a member of the electorate. Each ad hoc committee shall seek all appropriate consultation concerning the matters it is charged to study, including consultation with students enrolled in the School or house staff members. Ad hoc committees shall report their findings and recommendations to the Senate. An ad hoc committee is not necessarily dissolved at the end of the academic year in which formed, but continues its work until discharged by the Senate.

Article V: Committees of the Senate Pertaining to the Degree of Doctor of Medicine

Section 1

(1) The Committee on Medical Student Admissions (CA)

shall recommend to the Senate policies governing the admission of medical students, and together with the Dean and the Executive Committee of the School shall implement those policies adopted by the Senate. The CA shall make final decisions on the admission of applicants.

(2) The CA shall be composed of twelve voting members (including its chairperson). Ten shall be members (or emeriti members) of the electorate. Two members shall be medical students without current academic deficiency who have completed at least three clinical clerkships and who are eligible to fill a full term of service.

(3) The CA may enlist individual consultants or establish advisory panels to assist in the admissions process. These may include persons not members of the electorate.

(4) Six members of the CA shall constitute a quorum for any meeting of this committee.

Section 2

(1) The Committee on Medical Courses and Curriculum (CCC) shall recommend to the Senate policies concerning the curriculum of medical students and the criteria for their standing and promotion. It shall be the responsibility of the CCC, together with the Dean and the Executive Committee of the School, to implement those policies recommended by the CCC and adopted by the Senate.

(2) The CCC shall be composed of twelve voting members. Four shall be members of the electorate from the BMS Unit; four shall be members of the electorate from the Clinical Unit. The ninth shall be the Chairperson, from either Unit. The tenth and eleventh shall be medical students with one alternate, all without current academic deficiency. One student should be in his/her second year, and one must have completed at least two months of clinical clerkships.

Terms of service for each student is two years and the terms are staggered. The twelfth shall be the Senior Associate Dean for Education and Student Affairs, who shall serve also as executive secretary to the committee.

(3) The CCC may establish ad hoc advisory subcommittees to study particular issues. These may include students enrolled in the School, and other persons not members of the electorate.

(4) Seven members of the CCC shall constitute a quorum for any meeting of this committee.

Section 3

(1) The Committee on Medical Student Performance (CSP) shall consider and take action on matters that pertain to the meeting of the requirements for the MD degree by students in the MD programme, according to the policies adopted by the Senate and the criteria recommended by the CCC and adopted by the Senate; and it may also advise the CCC and the Senate concerning the criteria for student standing and promotion.

(2) The CSP shall be composed of five voting members, including its chairperson. The Assistant and Associate Deans for Student Affairs shall serve as ex officio nonvoting members. Voting members shall be members of the faculty of the School who have been members of the Faculty Council of the School of Medicine for at least the previous three years. Department chairpersons will be ineligible. An effort shall be made to have each department represented periodically. Three of the five members of the CSP shall be members of the Clinical Unit.

(3) The CSP shall formulate guidelines governing its procedures, and shall publish these in the School of Medicine Catalog. All changes shall be communicated to the Committee of Five before implementation. If, in the judgment of the

Committee of Five, a proposed change is significant enough to require approval by the Senate, implementation shall be withheld pending Senate approval. Changes considered not to require Senate approval shall nevertheless be communicated to the Senate at its next meeting.

(4) An affected student may appeal to the Dean from a final decision of the CSP. The Dean may affirm or overturn the decision of the CSP, or may refer the case back to the CSP for reconsideration.

Section 4

(1) The Medical Student Scholars Committee (MSSC) shall recommend to the Senate policies concerning the administration of medical scholars research fellowships. The MSSC, the Dean, and the Executive Committee of the School are responsible for implementing those policies recommended by the MSSC and adopted by the Senate. The MSSC shall make final decisions on the approval and disapproval of medical scholar fellowships to students.

(2) The MSSC shall be composed of ten voting members (including its chairperson). Four shall be members of the electorate from the BMS Unit; four shall be members of the electorate from the Clinical Unit. The ninth shall be an alumnus and the tenth shall be a medical student without current academic deficiency. The eleventh member shall be an Associate Dean for Student Affairs who is a nonvoting member.

(3) The MSSC may establish ad hoc subcommittees to assist in choosing students for the medical scholar fellowships. These may include students enrolled in the school, and other persons not members of the electorate.

(4) Six members of MSSC shall constitute a quorum for any meeting of this committee.

Article VI: Committees of the Senate Pertaining to the Degrees of Doctor of Philosophy & Master of Science

Section 1

(1) The Committee on Graduate Admissions and Policy (CGAP) shall recommend to the Senate policies governing the admission of graduate students, and together with the Dean and the Executive Committee of the School shall implement those policies adopted by the Senate. Each programme shall make decisions on the admission of applicants, using standards equivalent to or higher than those set by the Committee on Graduate Studies, a standing committee of the University Senate. The CGAP shall review and make final decisions on the admission of applicants to the graduate programmes in the School of Medicine.

(2) The CGAP shall be composed of seventeen voting members (including its chairperson). At least thirteen shall be members of the electorate from each of the graduate programmes in the School of Medicine, with two others from Biological Sciences and Biophysics. Two shall be graduate students without current academic deficiency who have completed at least their first year of graduate studies, and of these one shall be a member of the Biological Sciences or Biophysics programmes. The associate Deans for Graduate Education will serve as ex officio members and also as executive secretaries to the committee.

(3) The CGAP may enlist individual consultants or establish advisory panels to assist in the admissions process. These may include persons not members of the electorate and may be designated by each of the graduate programmes.

(4) Nine members of the CGAP shall constitute a quorum for any meeting of this committee.

Section 2

(1) The Committee on Graduate Curriculum (CGC) shall recommend to the Senate policies concerning the curriculum of graduate students and the criteria for their standing and promotion. It shall be the responsibility of the CGC, together with the Dean and the Executive Committee of the School, to implement those policies recommended by the CGC and adopted by the Senate with regard to graduate programmes in the School of Medicine.

(2) The CGC shall be composed of seventeen voting members. Thirteen shall be members of the electorate from each of the graduate programmes in the School of Medicine, and two shall be members of the programmes in Biological Sciences and in Biophysics. The sixteenth shall be the Chairperson, from any programme. The seventeenth shall be a graduate student with one alternate, each having completed at least two years in the graduate programmes, without current academic deficiency. The Associate Deans for Graduate Education will serve as ex officio members and as executive secretaries to the committee. The CGC shall work with graduate programme steering committees to develop optimum courses and curricula that meet the needs of all graduate students while making the most efficient use of faculty teaching resources.

(3) Graduate Programmes represented on this committee shall include Biochemistry, Cancer Biology, Developmental Biology, Epidemiology, Genetics, Health Research and Policy, Immunology, Medical Information Sciences, Microbiology and Immunology, Molecular and Cellular Physiology, Molecular Pharmacology, Neurosciences, and Structural Biology from the School of Medicine, along with Biological Sciences and Biophysics from the School of Humanities and Sciences.

(4) The CGC may establish ad hoc advisory subcommittees to study particular issues. These may include students enrolled in any of the affiliated graduate programmes, and other persons not members of the electorate. The latter could include faculty or others in other schools in the University as well as individuals, both alumni and others, affiliated with industry, government, and public and private foundations.

(5) Nine members of the CGC shall constitute a quorum for any meeting of this committee.

Section 3

(1) The Committee on Graduate Student Performance (CGSP) shall consider and take action on matters that pertain to the meeting of the requirements for the PhD and MS degree by students in those respective programmes, according to the policies adopted by the Senate and the criteria recommended by the CGC and adopted by the Senate; and it may also advise the CGC and the Senate concerning the criteria for student standing and promotion.

(2) The CGSP shall be composed of six voting members, including its chairperson. The Associate Deans for Graduate Student Affairs shall serve as ex officio nonvoting members and as executive secretaries. Voting members shall be members of the Faculty Council of the School of Medicine for at least the previous three years and shall be affiliated with one or more of the departmental or interdepartmental graduate programmes. Department chairpersons as well as directors of departmental or interdepartmental programmes will be ineligible. An effort shall be made to have each programme represented periodically. The CGC will work with each of the graduate programme steering committees in promoting adequate guidance, monitoring and counseling for all their graduate students.

(3) Graduate Programmes represented on this committee from time to time shall include Biochemistry, Cancer Biology, Developmental Biology, Epidemiology, Genetics, Health Research and Policy, Immunology, Medical Information Sciences, Microbiology and Immunology, Molecular and Cellular Physiology, Molecular Pharmacology, Neurosciences, and Structural Biology.

(4) The CGSP shall formulate guidelines governing its procedures, and shall publish these in the School of Medicine Catalog or on a specially designated Web site. All changes shall be communicated to the Committee of Five before implementation. If, in the judgment of the Committee of Five, a proposed change is significant enough to require approval by the Senate, implementation shall be withheld pending Senate approval. Changes considered not to require Senate approval shall nevertheless be communicated to the Senate at its next meeting.

(5) Matters referred to the CGSP will include decisions by the faculty of a graduate programme to suspend or dismiss a graduate student. An affected student may appeal an adverse action of the graduate programme to the CGSP. The CGSP may affirm or overturn the decision of the committee, or may refer the case back to the graduate programme for reconsideration. The affected student may also refer the affirmation of an adverse action by the CGSP to the Senior Associate Dean for Medical Education and Student Affairs and ultimately to the Dean.

Article VII: The Relationship between the Senate & the Electorate

Section 1

(1) Members of the electorate have the right to attend meetings of the Senate. Others may also attend unless the Senate decides otherwise on a particular occasion. Except

for Senators, the chairpersons of the standing committees, and the five nonvoting representatives specified in Article II, Section 4, (3), no one may participate in debate unless by permission of the Senate.

(2) All decisions of each meeting of the Senate, and the votes by which these decision were taken, shall be reported in writing to every member of the electorate within two weeks after the meeting.

Section 2

(1) Any decision of the Senate may be submitted to a meeting of the electorate by affirmative vote of forty percent of the membership of the Senate, or by petition of twenty percent of all members of the electorate to the Chairperson of the Senate. Notice and agenda of meetings of the electorate shall be sent to each member of the electorate by the Chairperson within one week of the vote in the Senate or of receipt of a petition, and this meeting shall take place not less than one week nor more than two weeks after dispatch of the notice. Seventeen members of the electorate shall constitute a quorum for a meeting of the electorate, and the Chairperson of the Senate or a delegate from among the Committee of Five shall preside at these meetings. Discussion at a meeting of the electorate shall be restricted to subjects germane to those specified in the notice and agenda convoking the meeting of the electorate.

(2) On request of forty percent of the membership of the Senate a mail referendum shall be submitted to each member of the electorate asking for approval or disapproval of the Senate decision specified in the referendum. The result of such a referendum shall be considered valid only if at least sixty percent of the members of the electorate vote.

(3) Decisions of the Senate may be confirmed, reversed,

or amended by majority vote at the meetings of the electorate or through the mail referendum, as specified in this Section (Article VII, Section 2). In any case, the Senate shall be free to take further decisions on the subject consistent with the vote of the electorate.

Section 3

(1) These Articles of Organization may be amended with the exception of those items noted in paragraph (2) of this Section either by a majority vote of the membership of the Senate concurred in by a meeting or mail ballot of the electorate, or by petition of twenty percent of the electorate concurred in by a meeting of the electorate, such meetings and mail ballots of the electorate being specified in Article VII, Section 2.

(2) In all matters relating to the role of the Dean or the Dean's designates or to the relationship of the Senate to the Executive Committee or to a change in the powers and function of the Senate, specifically including: Article I, Section 2; Article III, Section I, (1), (2) and (3) and Article V, Section 2, (1), any proposed amendments to these Articles of Organization shall be ratified by a majority of the membership of the Executive Committee of the School prior to their submission to the electorate. Such amendments shall take effect upon approval by the President of the University and the Board of Trustees.

APPENDIX TO THE ARTICLES OF ORGANIZATION FOR THE SENATE OF THE STANFORD UNIVERSITY SCHOOL OF MEDICINE FACULTY COUNCIL.

1. Standing Rules of the Senate

Provisions regarding governance of the Senate which do not require amendment of the Articles of Organization may be incorporated into these Standing Rules of the Senate.

2. Optional two-stage process.

A two-stage process for a decision by the Senate may be invoked subject to the following rules:

(a) The two-stage process for the consideration of a main motion may be invoked either (1) at the time of the introduction of the motion, on specification by the mover and seconder, or (2) during debate on the question, on motion from the floor, adopted by a majority vote.

(b) A motion to invoke the two-stage process is debatable with respect to the merits of invoking the process, requires a simple majority, and takes precedence over all other motions concerning the pending matter except a motion that a matter is not proper for official action by the Senate.

(c) Under the two-stage process, a preliminary vote may be taken on the question at the meeting at which the matter is introduced but such a vote shall in no respect be binding.

(d) A final vote on any matter being considered under the two-stage process shall be out of order on the same day as the preliminary vote is taken.

(e) After a preliminary vote, the matter involved shall be slated for final action no later than the next regular meeting in a position on the agenda outline which will assure its being considered at that meeting.

(f) During the second stage, secondary motions which are normally in order shall be applicable.

3. Procedure for preference voting.

(a) This method shall be used for the mail ballot to elect Departmental Senators and their alternates, Senators-at-Large and Alternates for Senators-at-

Large, the Chairperson of the Senate, and the remaining members of the Committee of Five.

(b) Each voter shall rank, in order of preference, a specified number of names. If the specified number is called N, then the highest preference shall be indicated by a preference score equal to N, and lower preferences by sequentially lower preference scores. If a voter fails to rank exactly N names, that ballot shall be disqualified.

(c) If a voter indicates a tied preference, the names so indicated shall receive the average of the preference scores they would have received had they not been tied, and lower choices on that ballot shall also receive the same preference scores they would have received had there been no ties in the list.

(d) Except as noted in 3 (b) above, a ballot shall be counted valid, even though the voter has failed to follow voting instructions literally, provided the voter's intent is clear and unequivocal.

(e) In the mail ballot to elect Senators-at-Large and Alternates for Senators-at-Large in each electoral unit, the specified number of names to be ranked shall be the total number of nominees in that electoral unit.

(f) In the election of Chairperson of the Senate, and in each election of the remaining members of the Committee of Five (two from among the BMS Senators, two from among the Clinical Senators), the specified number of names to be ranked shall be five.

(g) In counting the ballots, each candidate's total preference score shall be tabulated, and all names shall then be arranged according to total preference score, in a preference list. The positions shall be filled, in descending order, from the top of this preference list. In the election of Senators-at-Large and Alternates for Senators-at-Large, if a person who would otherwise be elected declines to serve, the person next lower on the preference list shall be elected. When all Senators-at-Large have thus been elected, in a given electoral unit, three names shall be chosen in the same manner and from the same preference list, to be Alternates for Senators-at-Large. The Alternate with the highest preference score in a given electoral unit shall be the First Alternate for that unit, and those with lower preference scores shall be designated Second Alternate and Third Alternate.

(h) Prior to the balloting by mail for selection of nominees for Chairperson of the Senate, and for the Committee of Five (Article III, Section 1, (1), eligible persons shall be given the opportunity to decline, and the names of such persons shall then be stricken from the list of the eligible.

(i) Whenever a tie will affect the outcome of an election, the tie shall be resolved by a special ballot in which the voters choose between the tied candidates.

4. Procedure for assuring attendance at the monthly meeting.

(a) Attendance will be taken for each meeting.

(b) Those senators who miss a meeting and have not notified their alternate will be contacted by phone by the Chairperson of the Senate or his or her designee to encourage their attendance at subsequent meetings.

(c) Those senators who miss two meetings and have not notified their alternate will receive a letter of reprimand from the Chairperson of the Senate.

REFERENCES

Balas EA, Boren SA, Brown GD, Ewigman BG, Mitchell JA, Perkoff GT. Effect of physician profiling on utilization. Meta-analysis of randomized clinical trials. *J Gen Intern Med* 1996; 11:584-90.

Bordley WC, Chelminski A, Margolis PA, Kraus R, Szilagyi PG, Vann JJ. The effect of audit and feedback on immunization delivery: a systematic review. *Am J Prev Med* 2000; 18:343-50.

Davis DA, Thomson MA, Oxman AD, Haynes RB. Changing physician performance. A systematic review of the effect of continuing medical education strategies. *JAMA* 1995; 274:700-5.

Dyer CC, Oles KS, Davis SW. The role of the pharmacist in a geriatric nursing home: a literature review. *Drug Intell Clin Pharm* 1984;18:428-433.

Folli HL, Poole RL, Benitz WE, Russo JC. Medication error prevention by clinical pharmacists in two children's hospitals. *Pediatrics* 1987;79:718-722.

Grimshaw JM, Russell IT. Effect of clinical guidelines on medical practice: a systematic review of rigorous evaluations. *Lancet* 1993; 342:1317-22.

Hatoum HT, Catizone C, Hutchinson RA, Purohit A. An eleven-year review of the pharmacy literature: documentation of the value and acceptance of clinical pharmacy. *Drug Intell Clin Pharm* 1986;20:33-48.

Jenkins MH, Bond CA. The impact of clinical pharmacists on psychiatric patients. *Pharmacotherapy* 1996;16:708-714.

Lesar TS, Briceland LL, Delcoure K, Parmalee JC, Masta-Gornic V, Pohl H. Medication prescribing errors in a teaching hospital. *JAMA* 1990;263:2329-2334.

Oxman AD, Thomson MA, Davis DA, Haynes RB. No magic bullets: a systematic review of 102 trials of interventions to improve professional practice. *CMAJ* 1995; 153:1423-31.

Szilagyi PG, Bordley C, Vann JC, Chelminski A, Kraus RM, Margolis PA, et al. Effect of patient reminder/recall interventions on immunization rates: A review. *JAMA* 2000; 284:1820-7.

Tett SE, Higgins GM, Armour CL. Impact of pharmacist interventions on medication management by the elderly: a review of the literature. *Ann Pharmacother* 1993;27:80-86.

Thomson O'Brien MA, Oxman AD, Davis DA, Haynes RB, Freemantle N, Harvey EL. Audit and feedback: effects on professional practice and health care outcomes. In: *The Cochrane Library*, Issue 2, 2000:Oxford: Update Software.

3

Hospital Staff Management: Select Case Study

IMPROVING INSTITUTIONAL PERFORMANCE BY BETTER INTERNAL HOSPITAL MANAGEMENT: A FRAMEWORK FOR ASSESSING MANAGEMENT TRAINING NEEDS

In the face of diverse contexts in the world's regions and countries, decentralization and increasing autonomy of hospitals are an important trend in hospital sector development. Substantial gains in institutional performance can be achieved through better internal hospital management. The article examines hospital managers' functions and practices and outlines a framework for assessing their management education needs. We argue that training is most appropriate if targeted at improving managerial competence within a specific health system development context. Enhancing a health system's performance (defined as the extent to which the system achieves its fundamental goals) is becoming a crucial concern for countries. The World Health Organization has responded to this challenge by developing a framework for performance assessment and improvement, delineated in the World health report 2000 and taken forward by a number of subsequent activities. The central emerging concept is an outcome-oriented approach to improving overall health system performance. More than a decade ago, WHO emphasized the need to strengthen the management of health services as one of the most crucial factors in bridging the gap between policy and implementation. Since then, important attempts at reform have been made in health systems around the world to increase the population's coverage with essential health interventions and to address key challenges in improving quality and efficiency of health care services and access to them. But setbacks in management of the services remain an acute issue. Managers face ever-increasing pressures imposed by recent trends such as decentralization and institutional autonomy, increased market exposure and new forms of public/private relationships in the health sector.

The contribution of internal hospital management to better hospital performance must be better understood. Issues to be examined include: the profiles of hospital managers in different settings; their functions and daily practices; the knowledge and skills they possess; and the support required to perform effectively. Special attention should be given to identifying opportunities to augment the managers' workplace competence by means of improved management education and training. To address the issue successfully, it is important to systematically analyse and comprehend the current context and challenges faced by hospitals. Most studies on internal hospital management come from the industrialized world. Little of this evidence is applicable to less-developed countries, and external assistance projects in the hospital sector there have a clear "macro" focus; institutional management issues are largely overlooked or are at best touched upon by vague recommendations to governments "to improve the managerial capacities" and/or by sporadic and very basic, short training events.

CASE STUDY: STAFF MANAGEMENT IN UK HOSPITALS

The two key areas that managers have to be concerned with in their job roles are managing their staff and managing the machines and tech-nology with which those staff have to work in order to do their jobs efficiently and effectively. How managers can, and should, relate to these two main areas of their work has been the concern of Robert Blake and Jane Mouton in their work on *The Managerial Grid.* This is a device for representing the concern for production and for people shown by different managers with a 1-9 scale being used to represent the degree of concern, 9 representing high concern.

Position 9,1: Efficiency in operations results from arranging conditions of work in such a way that human elements interfere to a minimum degree, by being concerned with acquiring the latest and most efficient technology which itself strictly controls the human input into the work process. This approach may well lead to staff frustration and demo-tivation through a lack of job satisfaction in feeling themselves to be essentially machine feeders and machine minders.

Position 1,9: This is the opposite approach, where the thoughtful attention of the manager to the needs of his staff for satisfying relationships leads to a comfortable, friendly organization atmosphere and working tempo, but, whilst job satisfaction and morale may be high, production may well not be as efficient as it could and should be. The danger is that more ruthless employers and managers of the 9,1 type will produce the same work at a quicker rate and lower cost and that the pleasant, cushioned surroundings created by the 1,9 manager will only be short-term before bankruptcy and redundancy take place.

Position 1,1: This is the least satisfactory approach of all, where the manager puts in the least effort possible, both with regard to his staff and production equipment in order to get the required work done and to sustain organization membership. The aim is purely to keep things ticking over to survive—a minimalist approach. In this situation, both the morale of the staff and the output of work is likely to be low and inefficient, leading to the twin problems of low motivation and uncom-petitive production.

Position 5,5: This is where an adequate level of performance is achieved through balancing the necessity to get the work out at a level of speed and efficiency which is competitive enough to provide an adequate level of profit, together with the desire to maintain the morale of the staff at a satisfactory level. It could be argued that this is the 'satisficing' level suggested by Herbert Simon.

Position 9,9: This is the optimum management approach, where work output and accomplishment is achieved through committed, highly-motivated staff who agree with, and believe in, the equal commitment to using the most efficient and productive technology available in order to be as competitive as possible. The management's attitude to the staff is that they are as important in the production process as the latest technology they work efficiently with, and this also creates an interdependence between management and staff through their feeling of having a 'common stake' in the purpose, objectives and methods of the organization, which leads to relationships of trust and respect.

It may be that some readers, particularly those who have always been employed in the NHS, will even now be shuddering at the mention of 'profit' in a book on health care management. Blake and Mouton are mainly concerned with profit-orientated commercial organizations. However, the current emphasis on privatization and the increasing use of performance indicators, should leave nobody in any doubt that even a relatively low-key interpretation of the word 'profit', as the most efficient and effective use of staff time and equipment to give the most cost-effective return on the upwards of £17 billion being annually pumped into the NHS should now be on all competent health care managers' lips. Although the Managerial Grid could be criticized as being somewhat simplistic, it could be argued that the gamut of specialist management books published each year could do with more simple, easily understood concepts and we feel the Grid is an excellent means of illustrating the balance in outlook and concern that each manager has to have between concern for his staff and concern for high-powered, efficient technology.

PEOPLE LEADERSHIP

One of the current areas of concern in the management literature is whether organizations tend to be over-managed and under-led. It could be argued that this is an extension of the other question of whether there is a difference between administrators and managers. The answer is that there certainly should be, as has been argued by Rosemary Stewart in the short-lived *Health Service Week* particu-larly in the restructured post-Griffiths NHS. The disturbing point is that, as the collated figures on district and regional general manager appointments have shown, 80% of these 'new appointments' come directly from the ranks of the ex-administrators. As a result of the implementation of Griffiths, the Institute of Health Service Adminis-trators has changed its name to the Institute of Health Service Management, which may be justified if there is, truly, a freeing and dynamization of these individuals from the normal role of adminis-trators, of the 'eminence grise' interpreter and manipulator of received rules, to the initiative-taking, policy-creating, decision-making role of management. Hopefully, fears that they may have changed the name, but will remain the same, will not be proved correct. Bennis and Nanus argue that there is a lack of leadership in many organizations and that they tend to be over-managed and under-led. They cite the case of Lee lacocca at Chrysler, who has become something of a modern management guru through his own writings,and led Chrysler from bankruptcy to success through his ability to handle properly the power he was given and mobilize successfully the employees behind his vision. He had the charismatic leadership qual-ities which perhaps should be looked for, but should probably be expected in smaller degrees at all levels of management in health care, from the chairman of the management board down to unit and sub-unit level management. The need for managers to have leadership qualities and what those should be in terms of effective person management has been well argued by John Adair. He suggests that there are three areas of leadership required within any given work group:

1. The need to accomplish the common task;
2. The need to maintain the team as a cohesive social unit;
3. The need to take account of the individual needs of group members.

The value of Adair's three overlapping circles is that they emphasize the essential unity of leadership functions and actions. A single action can be multi-functional in that it touches all three areas. He suggests a single list of leadership functions which managers need to follow to cater fully for all the areas:

1. *Planning:* seeking all available information. Defining the group task, purpose or goal. Making a workable plan in

the right decision-making framework; in his Training for Decisions' manual he clearly shows how this framework should be achieved by identifying, defining and analysing the problem, using imagination and brainstorming techniques to create all the possible solutions, and then analysing and choosing which is the optimum solution.

2. *Initiating:* briefing the work group on the aims and the plan. Explaining why the aim or plan is necessary. Allocating tasks to the group members. Setting group standards.

3. *Controlling:* maintaining group standards and influencing tempo. Ensuring all actions are taken towards the identified objectives. Keep-ing discussion relevant. Prodding the group to take action or to make new decisions.

4. *Supporting:* expressing acceptance of persons and their contri-bution. Encouraging the group/individuals. Disciplining the group/ individuals. Creating team spirit. Relieving tension with humour, humour being a most valuable management skill, and reconciling disagreements or getting others to explore them.

5. *Informing:* clarifying the task and the plan. Giving new infor-mation to the group, and keeping it 'in the picture'. Receiving information from the group and summarizing suggestions and ideas coherently.

6. *Evaluating:* checking the feasibility of an idea and testing the consequences of a proposed solution. Evaluating group performance. Helping the group to evaluate its own performance standards.

The way in which the leader or manager carries out these tasks will depend on four main variables:

1. The work situation, particularly the nature of the task and the time available for the decision;

2. The work group members, especially their attitudes, knowledge and experience;
3. The personality of the leader, introvert/extrovert, strengths/ weaknesses, values and attitudes.
4. The particular organization, its philosophy and values, structure, rules and objectives, its overall culture (as is well discussed by Handy), whether person, power, task or role culture.

The most effective group or team size is something which is also discussed by Handy, who suggests between 5 and 7 persons and Mintzberg, who is keen on groups of 5, for effectiveness. Certainly, 5 seems the best from our observation of the case-study teams dealing with management problems on the courses we run. It enables all members to have an effective influence in discussion—it appears much easier for individuals to become isolated and less involved in larger groups. As to the ideal characters of the personalities in a team for effective performance, this has been most interestingly studied by Meredith Belbin who suggests that a variety of characters is best for the most effective group decision-making; the chairman, the shaper, the company worker, the resource investigator, the plant, the monitor evaluator, the team worker and the finisher. This suggests an 8-person team is needed, but as Belbin points out, more than one role can be played by each individual within the group.

Communication

Fayol argues that a major management task is co-ordination, which means ensuring that one section's efforts are coincident with the efforts of other sections, which emphasizes the need for an overall departmen-tal manager, e.g. principal MLSO, superintendent radiographer, to be in charge of a whole area of health care work to provide an overall focus. There is a need to keep all activities in perspective with regard to the overall aims of the organization. Fayol felt this can only be achieved by a constant circulation of information and regular meetings of management which should lead to a binding together, unifying and harmonizing of all activity and effort. In another of his general principles of management, he argues that a hierarchy is necessary for unity of direction but that lateral communication is also fundamental as long as superiors know that such communication is taking place— this means the establishment of a cross-sectional and departmental matrix system of communication.

In well-run departments, there are three main types of communi-cation which managers and staff are daily involved in:

1. Written communications involving reports, circulars, and memos;
2. Verbal communication involving 'speeches', discussions, conver-sations, meetings;
3. Non-verbal communication involving dress, deportment, and physical and facial expression.

We would argue that managers should communicate with their staff as much as possible, to tell them what is happening, to ask their opinions and to involve them as much as possible in the work, so that they will self-manage themselves from a control point of view, and feel keen and willing to put up suggestions and new ideas from a planning point of view. Consultation is an important part of communication as the more that staff are consulted and feel trusted the better motivated they will be to do their best and make a positive contribution to their work.

Communications should be clear and precise to avoid

misinterpret-ation. As Lynda King Taylor says, 'If I were to choose just one failing which has done the most damage between employer and employee in the companies I have been involved with over the last ten years it would be the failure to communicate on easy terms... If communication is so simple, why do we not put it into simple words? If it is difficult, why cannot it be simplified? It has been the absence of simple communication and the inadequacy of the explanations and reasons for "change" which have helped cause the alienation now breeding in certain organizations, and these organizations are hoping to introduce new technology and systems within this kind of climate'. The truth of this is borne out by some of the events of the 1984/5 miners' strike and the introduction of new technology into *Times* newspapers. To persuade people of the need for, or advantages of, change, good communication is required. Communication is not one-way, from the manager down; it involves, in particular, the ability to listen to staff and to encourage reaction to statements and circulars, otherwise staff will become alienated and more likely to take disruptive or strike action. The need to develop an ability to listen carefully is vital for anyone hoping to become a really effective health-care manager. Chester Barnard has argued strongly that communication is necessary to translate purpose into action and that the ease and effectiveness of communication within a department and, therefore, the size of that department depends on:

1. The complexity of the purpose and the technological conditions for action;
2. The difficulty of the communication process, e.g. physical lay-out, noise;
3. The extent to which communication is necessary;
4. The complexity of the personal relationships involved.

The larger a department becomes, in terms of numbers of staff and physical size, the more difficult become the problems of effective communication. Barnard identifies, and stresses the importance of, the informal organization and its communication network which often exists within the formal organization and contributes vitally to its effective functioning. Managers need to be aware of, and to be able to use effectively, this 'grapevine' of communication within their health-care departments.

The Leader's Planning Role

The higher-level corporate planning function in health care has been looked at in the last chapter but the specialist departmental manager's role in having an upward say in the establishment of these plans as well as, perhaps, their key role in achieving their implementation at departmental level, needs to be emphasized here. There are four main areas of departmental planning—financial, production, manpower and sales and marketing—that health care managers have to be concerned with.

1. *Financial planning:* The health care leader/manager needs to plan carefully how much money he requires, in the form of a budget to run his department properly. It is vital that he has a say on the important committees deciding on budget allocations at regional, district and unit level, which under the current structure may be difficult, but which could be solved by the 'representative' structure of health care manage-ment that we have outlined. But whatever the formal budgeting structure is, all health care managers should establish at least informal links with their treasurer and finance officers, to ensure that the finance staff fully appreciate and understand their particular problems. It is useful to invite the treasurer to come and see and appreciate the work of each department. In order for the leader to

have a clear idea of departmental requirements it is important for him/her to consult all the section leaders and supervisory staff within the depart-ment so that all their financial needs are counted into the assessment of required resources. Both in putting forward a realistic claim and in planning expenditure within the given budget, which often, in practice, may be less than desired, it is necessary to assess and reassess working practices constantly to see if the scarce financial resources can be used in a more effective way through organizational or staffing changes. This will lead to:

2. *Production planning:* The manager will need to examine con-stantly the most effective use of technical and manpower resources. There is a need to keep constantly abreast of new technical develop-ments by attending exhibitions and demonstrations and talking to suppliers' sales staff, both to see and update knowledge of specialist departmental equipment and non-specialist computing systems.The manager will also need to examine the efficient use of staff resources in terms of their organization into rotas, on-call systems, or shift systems. This will lead to:

3. *Manpower planning:* Examining what type of staff are available and when to recruit, what training and retraining opportunities there are for them and what salaries and conditions to provide. These issues will be examined in detail later in this study. There is also, perhaps, the question of how most economically to shed staff.

4. *Planning sales and marketing:* It is important that the leader sells the importance of his department and the output and services it can provide both within the hospital and to the unit, district and regional management boards and health authorities. The manager's ability to do this may well have an important effect on his/her capacity to

obtain more funds, technical equipment improvements and more staff. It is vital to acquire the respect and support of the medical staff in this struggle for improved resources as they, naturally, have a great deal of influence and probably greater power than most health care staff. The priority in this 'sales' and 'marketing' should ultimately be to ensure that patients are given the best treatment.

We recognize that even the best treatment may, in some circumstances, be considered inferior to that offered by the private health care sector, particularly with respect to waiting lists, access to medical consultants and staff manning levels. The threat to the NHS from the private sector comes in two ways. First, a certain number of patients who can afford to do so are likely to take out private medical insurance and remove themselves from the NHS. Secondly, and more significantly, privatization of NHS services, in addition to cleaning, catering and laundering, is possible.

These could include, for example, clinical service functions such as pathol-ogy, particularly clinical chemistry and haematology, radiology and others. Whether this possibility is seen -as a threat or an opportunity will depend upon the attitude of individual managers and their staff. However, we believe that the desire and ability of health care managers to market and sell their services is generally, perhaps, greater now than it has ever been.

The importance of effective planning has been well emphasized by Henri Fayol, who feels that 'examining the future and drawing up a plan of action', prevoyance, is vital for good management and that planning should be an activity central to efficient management. He felt that the essence of planning was to allow the optimum use of resources which often, in the context of the NHS, are scarce resources. To function adequately, an organization and the specialist departments within it, need plans which are characterized by unity, continuity, flexibility and precision.

1. *Unity:* To make sure that the objectives of each part of the organization are securely welded together; this could apply to the NHS as a whole, the private hospital group as a whole, or the overall running of a specialist department, such as the pathology laboratory, to ensure that the individual specialisms of haematology, chemistry, microbiology and histopathology have a unity of approach and direc-tion. It may be best to have an overall manager drawn from the ranks of those doing the day-to-day work of the department, or a general manager, in order to provide a focus and catalyst to achieve unity. Whichever is considered better we would emphasize Fayol's principle of general management that an effectively run department must have unity of command with each person having only one boss and no other conflicting lines of command. The continuing battle between pro-fessional health care staff and medical consultant staff in some health care departments can be a major stumbling block to achieving this desired unity.

2. *Continuity:* By using both short-term and long-term forecasting.

3. *Flexibility:* Being able to adapt the plan in the light of changing circumstances. This is, perhaps, particularly important in the NHS, where sudden changes in the forecast RAWP allocations, as happened in January 1986, can have major effects on individual health care departments. Where regions find they are to get less or more money than expected in, say *3* months' time, the budgets of individual departments are required to be altered accordingly and often painfully for staff or patients if contraction is needed.

4. *Precision:* Attempting to predict courses of action

accurately, which, as indicated above, can be particularly difficult in the NHS.

As well as the importance of planning for good staff management, Fayol also emphasizes the need for good communication and motivation.

Meetings

The most commonly used form of management communication is through meetings and it is, therefore, essential that the meetings themselves are organized and managed effectively. Mintzberg has shown that 'the scheduled meeting consumes more of the manager's time than any other medium'. There are three main types of meeting which managers have to be involved in. These are:

1. Executive meetings, or what William Brown has called 'immediate-command' meetings where 'the manager calls the meet-ing at his own discretion, decides the procedure to be followed, and he alone is responsible for all the decisions taken';
2. Committee meetings, where the manager attends as a representa-tive of his department's interests and often, in health care, as a representative of his consumers' interests, often patients, but also general practitioners, and hospital medical staff;
3. Staff meetings, where issues affecting the department are opened up for all its members to discuss and give suggestions on and, on occasions, to make decisions about.

These three types of meeting fit in with Newman's three basic types:

1. Those in which decisions are finally taken or authorized by one particular person;

2. Those in which decisions are taken or authorized by the majority of the meeting;
3. Those in which decisions are taken or authorized only by unani-mous consent of those in the meeting.

It is likely that the executive meetings may well be *ad hoc* affairs, having to discuss issues and problems as and when they arise and. therefore, making the structured form of meeting with a properly compiled agenda difficult to achieve. However, firm controlled chair-manship is vital in all types of meeting. The major criticism that can be attached to meetings is their cost in terms of the salaried time of those attending, and so it is essential for the chairman to control the meeting so that as many participants as possible can contribute to the discussion. It may well be a good idea for the chairman to place a time-limit on the discussion of each agenda item so that the planned length of the meeting is not exceeded. It is important that Parkinson's 'law of triviality' is avoided where 'the time spent on any item of the agenda will be in inverse proportion to the sum of money involved' as well as his coefficient of inefficiency which would be a committee of more than 21 members. The other essentials for effective meetings are for dates and times to be fixed well in advance of the meeting, for the submission of agenda items and papers relating to those items, for circulation prior to the meeting, and for clear and accurate minutes of the proceedings to be taken.

Motivation

How far the manager will consult, and take account of, his subordinate managers' and his staffs ideas about issues, and the general organiza-tion and running of the department, will depend to a large extent on his/her own style and approach to the staff concerned. McGregor's classic text *The Human Side of the Enterprise* contrasted two sets of assumptions that managers tend to make about people:

1. Theory X—'the traditional view of direction and control.' This involved the assumptions that:

(a) The average human being has an inherent dislike of work and will avoid it if he can.

(b) Because of this human characteristic of dislike of work, most people must be coerced, controlled, directed or threatened with punishment, to get them to put forward adequate effort toward the achievement of organizational objectives.

(c) The average human being prefers to be directed, wishes to avoid responsibility, has relatively little ambition, wants security above all.

2. Theory Y—'the integration of individual and organizational goals'. The assumptions here are that:

(a) The expenditure of physical and mental effort in work is as natural as play or rest.

(b) External control and the threat of punishment are not the only means of bringing about effort toward organizational objec-tives. Man will exercise self-direction and self-control in the service of objectives to which he is committed.

(c) Commitment to objectives is a function of the rewards associated with their achievement.

(d) The average human being learns, under proper conditions, not only to accept but to seek responsibility.

(e) The capacity to exercise a relatively high degree of imagina-tion, ingenuity and creativity in the solution of organizational problems is widely, not narrowly, distributed in the popu-lation.

(f) Under the conditions of modern industrial life, the intellectual potentialities of the average human being are only partially utilized.

Although, at the time of writing his book, McGregor did not associate these sets of assumptions with managerial styles, Theory X has been widely assumed to equate with an 'authoritarian' style and Theory Y with a 'participative' style. The reality for most managers is likely to be that they recruit, or inherit, a mixture of both types of characters amongst their staff and that the art and science of staff management is to understand each person so as to know what kind of approach will result in achieving their best performance. It may, therefore, be that the skilled manager has to be capable both of being authoritarian in approaching some staff because they respond best to that approach, and participative in approaching others. It is likely, though, that the majority of skilled professionals employed in health care will be more responsive to the participative approach because of their generally high level of motivation to carry out the work they do. Tannenbaum and Schmidt have suggested a continuum of leader-ship behaviour ranging from 'boss-centred' to 'subordinate-centred', on which the following points are identified:

1. Manager makes a decision and announces it.
2. Manager 'sells' decision.
3. Manager presents ideas and invites questions.
4. Manager presents tentative decision subject to change.
5. Manager presents problem, gets suggestions, makes decision.
6. Manager defines limits; asks group to make a decision.

7. Manager permits subordinates to function within limits defined by him to make their own policy decisions.

In talking to groups of MLSOs and radiographers on management courses run by us, an approach somewhere between 5 and 6 is usually seen as the most suitable, generally, and this would seem to be the most likely successful approach for professional staff. The importance of supervisors and managers taking a personal interest in the performance of their staff has been illustrated by the somewhat dubious Hawthorne experiments. Although he did not con-duct them, his conclusions, published some time before the factual account of the experiments, assured Elton Mayo's place in history.as the founder of the Human Relations School of Management.

General experiments were conducted in the Western Electric Company in Chicago between 1927 and 1932. Initially, a group of manual assembly workers were subjected to different levels of illumination for their work. Their productivity rose as the lighting improved, but then (unexpectedly) continued to rise when it was severely reduced. Produc-tivity in the control group also rose! A later experiment extended variations to other working conditions such as rest pauses and pay. Similar findings resulted and Mayo attributed the rise in productivity, seemingly unrelated to working conditions, to the workers' interaction and co-operation being intensified, their informal practices, values, norms and social relationships being built up within the groups, giving high cohesion, as a result of the interest shown in these workers merely by conducting the experiments. This response has become known as the Hawthorne Effect. A critical evaluation of Mayo's work, and of the Hawthorne experiments, by Rose shows that as research these experiments were flawed. However, rightly or wrongly, Mayo's name is firmly associated with the Human Relations approach to management.

The relationship between motivation and the development of socially cohesive groups within the work organization has been illus-trated by Trist and Bamforth's work in the coal-mining industry for the Tavistock Institute of Human Relations. They found that the replacement of the small team approach of the existing short face method of extracting coal by the highly mechanized and innovative 'longwall' method had been introduced without consideration of its social consequences. This new method had a deleterious effect on morale and motivation and on sickness, accident rates, absenteeism and productivity. Following the introduction of the 'composite long-wall' method matters improved. Within the necessary technological and economic restraints which had been the major arguments for introducing the longwall technology the composite method enabled groups of men to be given responsibility for a whole task, to allocate themselves to shifts and to jobs within a shift, and to be paid on a group bonus basis; these all being traditional features of coal-mining. By this system, the problems of over-specialized work roles, segrega-tion of tasks across shifts with consequent scapegoating, and lack of group cohesion, were overcome.

A similar philosophy to increase motivation has been behind the attempts at Volvo in Sweden to improve the quality of working life of their staff by enabling production workers to be involved with the production of a whole car, rather than just doing one or two specific tasks, e.g. fitting engines, wheel-alignment or paint-spraying, and thus losing any sense of identity with, or responsibility for, the final product. This problem emanated from Henry Ford's invention of the car production line in 1913 and the problem of de-skilling and demotivation which it and later technological developments have brought to workforces has been interestingly examined by Braver-man. Fred Herzberg has been a prime mover in the effort to get managers to look at the problem of how jobs can be enriched to improve motivation. His work springs from his motivation-hygiene theory which resulted initially from a survey of 200 engineers and accountants representing a cross-section of Pittsburgh industry.

Collating the information based on 12 different investigations, involving over 1600 employees in a variety of jobs in business and other organizations, he has shown that the overwhelming majority ofthe factors contributing to job satisfaction—81 %—were the motiva-tors concerned with growth and development in the content of the job; whereas a large majority of the factors contributing to job dissatisfac-tion—69%—involved what he termed hygiene or environmental main-tenance. Herzberg advocates that those factors in the work setting which provide motivation, should be developed and concentrated upon to enrich jobs; these being the rewarding nature of the work itself, recognition, responsibility, and opportunities for achievement and advancement. If this is done, job satisfaction can be increased and staff effectively utilized. He therefore advocates an industrial engineer-ing approach, based on the design of jobs but from the opposite point of view to F. W. Taylor's 'scientific management' approach which aimed mainly at rationalizing and simplifying work to increase efficiency, rather than enriching it.

The principles of job enrichment require that the job be developed to include new aspects, which provide the opportunity for the employee's psychological growth, and aim to improve the dissatisfying 'hygiene' areas of work which he identifies as company policy, administration, technical supervision, salary, and interpersonal relationships.

Herzberg emphasizes that it is important that the new satisfying aspects are capable of providing enrichment—merely to add one undemanding job to another, as is often the case with job enlargement, or to switch from one undemanding job to another, as in job rotation, is not adequate. These are merely forms of horizontal job loading. Job enrichment calls for vertical job loading where opportunities for achievement, responsi-bility, recognition, growth and learning are designed into the job. There are numerous ways that this can be done, for example:

1. Removing some controls, while retaining or increasing an indi-vidual's accountability for his/her own work;
2. Giving a person a complete, natural, unit of work;
3. Granting additional authority to an employee in his/her job;
4. Increasing job freedom;
5. Making reports/minutes directly available to the staff themselves rather than just to the supervisor;
6. Introducing new and more difficult tasks not previously under-taken.

Herzberg argues that the more subordinates' jobs become enriched, the more superfluous does 'on the job' supervision become, and the more self-control and self-management are exercised. Managers' and supervisors' jobs are not down-graded by this process as, in the companies where he carried out his studies and introduced his ideas, they found themselves free to develop more important aspects of their jobs with a greater managerial component than before.

Managing people who have authority of their own is a more demanding, rewarding and enjoyable task than simply checking on the every move of circumscribed automatons.

Maslow's famous *Hierarchy of Needs,* whilst less well-researched than Herzberg's work, has drawn wide support and suggests there are various needs that all employees are seeking to satisfy from their work. Maslow's contention is that the lowest need requires satisfying before the one above it becomes important for an individual employee. He argues that the ultimate aim for all staff is to self-actualize but how far any one individual gets towards achieving this state depends partly on the culture of the organization, the management style of its managers, and the inherent ambition of the employee him/herself. Although employees would normally work their way up the needs pyramid and then not be concerned with the lower-level needs this will only be the case so long as these lower needs remain satisfactorily and adequately catered for. If, for instance, someone who had reached a position of autonomy was suddenly confronted with a move to a less modern and less pleasant building or site, then it is likely that his once satisfied physiological needs will again come back to the fore of his needs concerns. Alderfer has simplified the hierarchy to three cate-gories, Maslow's bottom two categories being termed existence needs, the middle two relatedness needs, and the top two growth needs.

The other key skill for both motivating staff and effectively running a department is the ability to delegate. Apart from being the skill that is most likely to prevent ill-health in the manager in the form of stress-related diseases, delegated responsibilities are most likely to inspire subordinates to feeling they are being trusted and relied upon, thus increasing their overall job satisfaction. It is important to bear inmind that anyone who has a responsibility delegated to them must also be given the requisite level of authority to carry the task out— responsibility without authority is likely to cause the subordinate great stress, and demotivation. A good delegator will ensure that subordi-nates do not suffer from role underload which can cause great boredom and which can be stressful, but a manager must ensure that he does not become a bad delegator by trying to off-load too much of his work onto a subordinate, thereby causing that person to suffer from very stressful role overload. Being a good delegator is not easy, as every manager has a tendency to want to say 'I' m the boss, I've got to make sure these tasks are done properly and the person I can best rely on is myself, so I'll do it.' There is also the problem that Handy terms the 'trust-control dilemma' which he described as 'the essence of the delegation problem. The dilemma is that in any one managerial situation the sum of trust plus control is always constant... The implications of this constant sum are that:

1. Any increase in the control exercised by the manager decreases the amount of trust perceived by the subordinate: control + x = trust — x.
2. Any wish by the manager to increase his trust in his subordinate, to give him more responsibility, must be accompanied by the release of some control if it is to be believed: trust + x = control — x.'

Getting this dilemma right lies at the heart of effective delegation, which itself lies at the heart of effective motivation. The effective management and motivation of staff is thus vital to being an efficient health care manager but, as has been pointed out, these features are dependent not only on personal management skills, but on the talents and abilities and approach of all staff. It is, therefore, vital that every manager develops good personnel management skills in the areas of manpower planning, recruiting, training, re-training, appraising staff and job evaluation, to ensure responsive staff who will link well with the manager's skills.

Personal Management

Alec Rodger, who was Professor of Occupational Psychology. at Birkbeck College, has highlighted the importance, and interlinking, of fitting the person to the job and fitting the job to the person, in all organizations. In personnel management, managers are mainly concerned with the upper hemisphere but also with rewards, compensation and incentives. The first concern should be manpower planning to make sure that there is an adequate supply of appropriately qualified and talented staff to carry out the work demands of the specific health care department which you are managing.

1. An evaluation of existing resources which is often referred to, as a 'Manpower Audit'. This is something that any newly appointed health care departmental manager should carry out on his appointment, particularly if he has been appointed from outside the department and has no knowledge of the existing staff. It is probably best achieved by a combination of looking at the existing staff records and carrying out a personal 'getting to know staff interview, in order to clarify what their qualifications, experience and aspirations are.

2. An assessment of the manpower requirements needed to achieve output and patient care objectives. This will indicate whether the department is adequately staffed to carry out the current workload and any future developments that are envisaged. This assessment needs to be carried out in tandem with an appraisal of work output and productivity in terms of the department's performance indicators.

3. Measures to ensure that the necessary resources are available when required. This will require lobbying the unit general manager and perhaps those of district and region to ensure that proper funding is made available for

adequate staffing. It is also vital for the health care manager to see that staff vacancies are, where appropriate, filled immediately they become vacant, in order to prevent overwork and stress for the remaining staff whilst a replacement is sought. It is something of a tragedy for efficient manpower planning that it has become virtually established financial practice to make savings on the annual staffing budget by not filling posts immediately, and allowing, say, a 3-month gap between a person leaving and another being recruited or, increasingly, freezing indefinitely posts that fall vacant. This can be very disruptive to the efficient running of health care departments, particularly if a disproportionate number of a particular health care staff group leave, thus causing one department to be far below adequate staffing levels. In an ideal world, the best form of manpower planning would be to have replacement staff engaged some time prior to the present job-holder leaving, in order to provide a change-over and run-in training period for the new member. This would again help the efficiency of the department, and help to reduce the time spent training new members of staff.

To achieve these objectives manpower planning involves ten basic activities:

(a) Defining the overall corporate objectives for the stated period ahead as expressed in the corporate plan. This would currently involve ensuring adequate manpower to provide health care services for the defined national priority areas within health care in the NHS, as well as the known district and regional requirements which might well impose specific disease demands on particular health care departments.

(b) Converting these corporate objectives into manpower

objectives for the same period, allowing for changes in productivity, methods used, and product mix. An essential part of manpower planning is equipment and machine planning to see if a more effective and efficient, and less costly, service can be provided by investing in new technology. This is particularly important when, as in the health service, staff costs and salaries account for about 75% of the total expenditure on the service.

(c) Designing a manpower information system including potential sources of manpower, e.g. schools, colleges, universities, and an effective record system for current staff.

(d) Undertaking a manpower inventory, looking at the composition of the staff and how they are deployed and utilized.

(e) Analysing manpower requirements in terms of jobs to be done; roles to be carried out; the type of new staff required to be recruited, i.e. graduates or non-graduates; particular areas of experience required; and the requirements of existing staff in terms of develop-ment through training and re-training courses, both within the depart-ment and at outside educational establishments.

(f) Analysing manpower supply in terms both of the staff already employed in the department and their skills, talents and abilities, and suitability for promotion, and staff available outside the department, both new recruits from schools, colleges, universities, and trainees and experienced staff employed in similar health care departments in other hospitals, who might be looking for a sideways move or promotion.

(g) Improving manpower utilization which should be relatively simple after completing *(a)* to (f).

(h) Improving manpower policies within the health care departments which, again, should follow from the above actions, but this process should also influence the whole unit to examine thoroughly its man-power planning procedures in all departments, from portering to medical manpower.

(i) Identifying training needs and an assessment of training effective-ness for both trainee and experienced staff, both internally and externally.

(j) Controlling manpower costs—as with management generally, planning and control are inextricably linked, and thus the whole formalization and tightening up of effective staff planning should lead to a more efficient use of staff resources and training and thus greater control of manpower costs.

Recruitment

Once a proper manpower plan has been established, then it needs to be applied to the recruitment policy for employing new staff. The vital importance of 'fitting the person to the job' and 'fitting the job to the person' has already been illustrated in the adaptation of Alec Rodger's model for the effective use of manpower. Probably the most vital task is that of personnel selection, since if the calibre, quality and potential for development of those recruited is poor then any organization or department within an organization is storing up untold future problems for itself. It is vital to establish an efficient procedure for attracting the right people to apply for vacan-cies and then to find an effective means of obtaining a true impression of their talents and abilities and forming a judgement as to whom to select.

The first essential is to carry out a job analysis to establish what the key criteria are for performing the particular job well, and from this to draw up a 'person description' of the most suitable temperament, skills and abilities required to perform the job effectively and to fit in with the culture and personalities of the department doing the recruitment.

The first stage, therefore, involves a careful study of the duties, responsibilities, and requirements of the job to be filled, and an assessment of the relevant personal characteristics deemed necessary for successful performance. These would include such features as general education, specific training, type and depth of experience, analytical ability, social skills, psycho-motor skills, written and verbal powers of communication, numerical ability, powers of comprehen-sion and judgement, personality factors relating to adaptability and acceptability, and attitudes to authority and responsibility.

A very useful means of formulating these criteria can be obtained by analysing the most commonly reported 'difficulties' and 'distastes' occurring in the particular job to be advertised or a closely similar job. These two critical variables will give clues as to the main capacities needed for successful performance of the job, and the personal inclinations which have a bearing both on performance and job satisfaction. The precise details of the duties and responsibilities should be written up in a Job Description and the personal qualities necessary should be specified in a Job Specification. Both documents should lack ambiguity, be concise statements of crucial elements in the job and be the subject of consensual agreement between line management, the personnel depart-ment or job analyst, and, where possible, other similar job holders, since they should have a better idea than anyone of the skills, abilities and personality required to do the job well.

It may well be the case that personnel departments within the health service should be more involved in the recruitment of health care professionals than they currently are. Once they are qualified and experienced, personnel assistants will be a valuable asset to the specific health care departments in helping to draw up accurate and effective descriptions and specifications by providing a detached, objective viewpoint. They obviously need to prove their value in this advisory role and line management must give them a proper opportunity to provide it. Once this job analysis has been carried out, then recruit-ment advertisements need to be placed in the most appropriate professional journals and newspapers.

The most appropriate publi-cation will obviously depend on the level of the job, and the experience and qualifications required to perform it. The advertisement itself should contain as much information as space and cost permit in order that a certain amount of self-selection can take place in the target population. It is perhaps too simplistic to say, as the DHSS has recently done, that costs in this area must be reduced, without giving due consideration to the potentially far higher costs of advertisements which do not give enough information for self-selection to take place properly.

This can lead to a large expenditure of staff time on sending application forms and sifting them, as well as endless informal visits. The advertisements also have to be distinctive and attractive in a competitive market and there has been a certain amount of criticism that individuality and personality in job advertisements has been lost by the current DHSS rules. The most important aspect, though, is that the advertisement must be placed in the most appropriate media for the type and level of post concerned and this decision is probably best left to the health care management professionals themselves.

The application forms which are sent to candidates need to be properly structured and designed to elicit pertinent, non-trivial infor-mation about an applicant's attributes and autobiographical detail. It is debatable whether the increasing fashion for candidates to submitcurriculum vitae is better than the form, as standard forms make cross-comparisons between candidates easier than c.v.s, which may be non-standard and may not concentrate on the areas which the employer is most concerned with. However, c.v.s give scope for initiative, imagina-tion and self-expression often inhibited by the application form.

Shortlisting will normally take place on the basis of the applications received, but the health service has in a number of health care areas encouraged the practice of candidates attending for an 'informal visit'. This is obviously very valuable in that it gives both the candidate and the recruiting department the opportunity to assess each other. The major criticism of the current system is that candidates are expected to take time off and pay their own fares to attend such visits. Obviously, this can be a useful measure of their keenness and interest in a particular vacancy, but there is a limit to an individual's desire to lose holiday and to self-finance what may be expensive trips.

In the current climate of financial strictures on health authorities there may anyway be a tendency for the local candidate to be favoured, perhaps due to the high cost of transfer, particularly to South-East England. Thus a perfectly good candidate may omit such visits and a department may lose the opportunity of recruiting valuable external 'new blood', simply because this particular 'hurdle' has not been jumped. To avoid this potential problem, perhaps it would be better for the 10 best candi-dates on paper to be asked to an informal visit, for which expenses would be paid by the employing authority, and time off would be allowed, and then a shortlist could be drawn up from those attending. In other words, a two-stage interview would become the norm. Once a shortlist has been drawn up it is vital to notify both the successful and unsuccessful candidates as soon as possible unless you have previously stated that if candidates do not hear within a certain time period they should assume that they have been unsuccessful. This is another way of reducing costs, as is the practice of asking candidates to send a stamped, addressed envelope for an application form and further details of the job. However, it is questionable what this practice does to the candidate's perception of their potential employer and whether it does not give the impression of a somewhat overbearing financial structure and, indeed, put them off applying, as with the practice of the informal visit.

The successful candidates need to be given the time and place to attend the recruitment process which still, often, takes the form of a single interview by a panel of interviewers. Although the interview process has been criticized from time to time, it has survived, in the words of the eminent Professor of Occupational Psychology at Birkbeck College in the 1950s and 1960s, Alec Rodger, 'because the interview is a widely accepted technique of assessment, and is likely to remain so. The main task of the psychologist in this field is, while pursuing his attempts to devise satisfactory objective means of assess-ment to do his best to find out where interview judgements go wrong and to remove their defects. In a word, his business is not to disparage the interview, but to improve it'. Rowan Bayne of the Civil Service Behavioural Science Unit has agreed in stating that 'interviewing is a very high-level skill which has been ill-treated and taken for granted, and in the variety of interviews and interviewers lies the possibility of sufficient improvements'.

Whilst agreeing with these statements and feeling that the attitude 'anyone can interview' is a dangerous and too often present attitude amongst many senior staff, not only in the health service, it may also be true that practical, objective tests of candidates' ability are not used as often or as widely as they might be, particularly in some of the health care professions where manual dexterity, hand-eye co-ordination, and practical skill are vitally important. This is particularly true at the less senior levels where the major part of the staffs work involves practical as well as mental skills. If there are objective tests which can be developed to back up interview assessments then it is vital that they should be used.

In order for the interviewing process to be improved, Bayne has made a number of proposals. Firstly, interviewers need to have a prepared 'state of conciousness' at the interview and he suggests that the 'calm-alert' state, where the 'interviewer's calmness helps the candidate to relax and his or her clear perception allows productive silences and the easy asking of questions' is what should be aimed for. Ways of achieving this state include meditation and some mental exercises. Perhaps mass recruitment panel yoga on the day of the interview would be taking this suggestion too far, but how often have managers arrived for an interview in a rushed and hurried frame of mind thinking more of the day's other problems rather than the interview to come?

Some kind of immediate pre-interview meeting is essential in order to clarify what qualities are being looked for, to decide on what questions are to be asked, and who should ask them. Secondly, there is a need to make sure that 'good interviewers' are involved who have either had training in good techniques or have the right personalities or states of consciousness for the role. Bayne defines these as 'calm, alert, warm, interested, analytical and perceptive'. He also suggests that the right 'voice quality' may be important, and that training should be given to interviewers to ensure that their voice tone and pitch draws out the best response from the candidate by the way in which the interview questions are asked. Thirdly, the social and physical contexts need to be considered. Should there be one 'panel' interview or a series of interviews with different people? Panels have the disadvantage of inducing inhibition in candidates, but the countering advantage of providing a varied view in deciding whom to select.

It is important that the right people are on the panel and that the manager most directly concerned with the day-to-day work of the candidate should have the greatest say and probably chair the proceedings.

There is a problem in the health care profession with some medical consultants wishing to be a panel member for quite junior appointments, in pathology and radiology particularly, which is probably an unnecessary waste of what should be valuable time. As head of department, they could appropriately delegate such responsibility. They will obviously want to play a role in the appointment of more senior staff, but this should normally be as a member of the panel with one voice in the decision, a more dominant role might be expected where an immediate subordinate was being appointed. The personnel department should play an important advis-ory role in the conduct of the interviews, and act as the organizers and chair of the pre-interview panel meeting, as well as an active one during the interview.

An experienced personnel officer can contribute much to the inter-view, by giving a different angle to questioning and by analysing the candidates responses. As far as is possible, the personnel office will advise on problems of employment law and seek to prevent panel members asking 'discriminatory' questions. His/her notes of the inter-view, its outcome and the reasons for that outcome are retained by the personnel department for reference in cases of enquiry or complaint. In addition to explaining salary and conditions of service, personnel officers may also spot weaknesses in interviewing technique and identify possible training needs.

The physical location for the interview is important and this should ideally be in a comfortable, self-contained area away from noise and interruptions, where the candidates can wait in comfort and get refreshments. The seating in the interview room should be as comfor-table as possible and efforts should be made to ensure that it is arranged in order to make verbal interaction with the candidate as easy as possible. Attention should also be paid to the installation of pleasant lighting and furnishings which will help to put the candidates at ease in what is always a stressful situation. It is important to have a means for recording information given during the interview, and for the members of the panel to assess candidates individually, as the interview is taking place. There are popular models, such as Alec Rodger's 7-Point Plan or the Munro Fraser 5-Point Plan, which examine a candidate's impact on others, his/her qualifications or acquired knowledge, innate abilities, motivation and emotional adjustment or ability to cope with stress.

Job Evaluation

The other important element in being able to recruit the right people is the level of pay offered for the work required. The problem the Health Service has lies in its established incremental pay rates which are extremely rigid in their operation. All large organizations need to establish an agreed salary band for a particular job and if this is done properly by agreed, jointly carried out procedures involving both staff and management, as should be done in the best form of job evaluation system, then they should be adequate to attract the right calibre of staff into a profession and, indeed, to persuade students to enter into training for a particular profession. Part of the reason for the great demand for places on medical courses at university, apart from the intrinsic interest of the work itself, is undoubtedly the excellent financial rewards that are achievable at GP or consultant level.

The difficulty the Health Service has is that, because of agreed Whitley rules, there is little flexibility in the incremental point on a particular scale that an individual can be offered initially, and because there is no performance appraisal system, there is also no scope for staff to obtain additional incremental awards for particularly proficient performance, which happens in many large private sector organizations. As well as the rigidity of the pay rates, many might also argue that they are inadequate and unfair in their differentials between the various groups of health care professionals and, indeed, that such differentials are extremely hard to justify if one uses as a major criterion of evaluation the value of the particular profession's work to the actual eventual return to good health of the patient. This problem of pay has been looked at in three reports of the National Association of Health Authorities, working in conjunction with the King's Fund. However, whilst carrying out a useful analysis of comparative pay levels in the NHS and suggesting a new overall NHS payment system, these reports, surprisingly to these authors, come out against a complete job evaluation of all health care groups, even though one of their four criteria for producing an orderly and acceptable pay system is that 'it should be flexible enough to attract sufficient staff of the necessary quality to achieve perceived national and local service needs and objectives'. They argue against a complete job evaluation '... for three reasons. First, the evaluation would be a lengthy affair which would hold up necessary change. Second, the changing nature of many jobs in the health service would make such an evaluation out-of-date almost before completion ... our third reason ... is because the costs need to be clearly identified and budgeted for.' The problems with these arguments are that, firstly, how lengthy a full evaluation would be is debatable, and it could well be that an experienced firm of manage-ment consultants would be able to carry out such an evaluation within a year, so that necessary change need not be 'held up'. Even if this was not possible, one of the major problems of the management of change is often undue haste, rather than gradually gaining the staffs support and acceptance, which should be an important part of any well-conducted evaluation.

It is doubtful if the essential characteristics of the vast majority of jobs in the health service change as rapidly as is suggested and, anyway, once a proper cross-profession evaluation study has been conducted and agreed, then enhanced duties and responsibilities could be rewarded by moving staff to a higher estab-lished scale if their duties had changed so dramatically. The third criticism is hard to understand since a tender for conducting the evaluation could be put out to a number of consultancies, and so the cost would be known before it was conducted and could therefore be budgeted for within NHS resources—it is not beyond the bounds of possibility that some or all of the cost could be provided by agreement between the NHS representative bodies and the government to fund it out of the annual sum available for pay increases. This would only be achievable if the government gave a commitment to enact and fund the evaluation's eventual findings which might, of course, be expensive.

The problem with the NAHA/King's Fund proposals for a new salary structure is that they are an arbitrary stab at a solution— undoubtedly a conscientious, analytical stab— by a group of well-qualified people, but it goes against the first rule of a proper job-evaluation scheme which is the establishment of democratically consti-tuted committees of management and employees, as well as the personnel department and management consultants, if they are involved.

An alternative to the expense of employing consultants would be for the management board personnel director to use the personnel staff resources available within the NHS to instigate an internal job-evaluation review. Whatever means is used, a series of consultative, democratic committees should be established to evaluate the work of all the health care professions, and to see if some common scales could be established. Such a review would need to encompass all terms and conditions of employment, as these would need to be standardized in all areas (i.e. hours and holidays, whether 'on-call' duties are compulsory or voluntary), to fit in with a standardized reward system.

The committees would need to establish 'benchmark' jobs, anchor-age points around which to make qualitative and quantitative judge-ments of other jobs, in terms of such factors as qualifications, training, skill, effort, responsibility and working conditions. A points analysis would be carried out for each factor analysed in each job and once a ranking had been established, between health care professions, and between grades of jobs in each profession, then salary ranges would be established and broken down into incremental points.

The points value placed on jobs must relate solely to the work and the responsibilities involved in it, and must ignore any favourable or unfavourable personal aspects of the current job-holder which might give a 'halo' or other effect to the assessment of the job itself. Another criticism of the NAHA/King's Fund proposed reform is that there are only 3 or 4 increments in each grade which is probably too limited for incentive purposes, when one takes account of the disincentive problem of staff feeling they are stuck at the top of a grade, and 8-10 incremental points would probably be a better structure. This number also gives some room for extra merit increments in an appraisal system, if such a system is introduced into the NHS.

Elliott Jacques has written widely on this subject and believes that an individual's capacity for work, the work actually done and the payment received, should be in equilibrium, C-W-P, otherwise staff will feel overstressed or underpushed, and that this equilibrium can be greatly helped by a job evaluation system. He propounds the idea that 'there exists an unrecognized system of norms of fair payment for any given level of work, unconscious knowledge of these norms being shared among the population engaged in employment work' and that 'an individual is unconsciously aware of his own capacity for work, as well as the equitable pay level for that work'. Thus, to be equitable, pay must be felt to match the level of work and the capacity of the individual to do it—the 'felt-fair' principle which can be achieved by job evaluation schemes.

One of the major problems that the NAHA/King's Fund report and some of the other articles in the Health Service Journal confront is the need for whatever scales are decided upon to contain flexibility so that local difficulties relating to the demand for, and supply of, particular health care skills, can be compensated for by offering higher local rates of pay to those groups where there are shortages. Whether this is really feasible within a 'National' health service, is debatable, but a cental objective of the job evaluation procedures that we feel is vital for the health service to carry out would be to introduce greater flexibility and, indeed, greater rationality, into the payment and grading systems of individual health care groups. One only has to look at the incremental scales for MLSOs to see some of the quirks and problems of the present system where incremental rises are irregular and often quite small, and the principal grade only has two incremen-tal points—a job evaluator's nightmare!

Interview Strategy

It is best to:

1. Begin on an easily conversable topic, maybe some past achieve-ment reported in the application form, in order to establish a measure of confidence and rapport with the candidate.
2. Avoid leading questions such as, 'You are a member of the Conservative Party?', which indicates the reply you want and expect, as any intelligent candidate will give the desired response, and such questions do not glean any valuable information.
3. Ask open-ended questions which require more than monosylla-bic 'yes/no' answers. This is likely to assist and encourage the candi-date to speak with greater freedom and will, therefore, reveal more information on which to base the assessment.
4. Follow the interviewee's lead wherever possible, whilst keeping to the areas you want to find out

about and enquire into, and without straying into irrelevant areas such as, for example, descriptions of last year's walking holiday.

5. There is a need to check the validity of responses by an interrogatory style, probing in depth relevant areas of experience, looking for traits of marked generality, consistency and persistence.
6. Avoid trick questions designed to reveal inconsistencies as they only foster antagonism.
7. Hold back difficult questions until later in the interview, when rapport has been established.
8. Do not: reveal your reactions; make moral judgements; reveal your own biases and prejudices; interrupt a candidate in full flow unless he/she is going off the point or talking about something irrelevant; be loquacious—interview panels should not be the location for personal ego trips for panel members.
9. Listen very carefully to everything that is said and give your undivided attention to the proceedings, even when boring.
10. Pay particular attention to a candidate's revealed or underlying 'difficulties' and 'distastes', and the capacities and inclinations which his/her record and general impression indicate to be his/her relative strengths and weaknesses for overcoming them. There is a need to observe and interpret facial expressions and bodily movement for signs of dissonance, which may indicate an attempt to cover over problems previously experienced.
11. Give the candidate a full and fair hearing, making sure the interview plan is fully covered, and ensuring that you have enough information about the

candidate on which to make comparative decisions *vis-d-vis* the other candidates.

12. It is vitally important not to be swayed either by a candidate's appearance 'looks smart, therefore must be smarter than he seemed' or by some halo effect 'went to my old university, must be an intelligent person even though she didn't come across well—nervous' which could illogically sway your judgement of a candidate.
13. Arriving at sound judgements and discriminating fairly between individuals is probably the most difficult task of all. Inferences must be drawn from the evidence as presented. Expertise in this area is partly intuitive, partly due to training, practice and experience, but, in all cases, considerably enhanced by careful preparation and professional conduct.
14. Inform the candidates of the outcome as soon as possible, decisions are normally taken on the day of the interview, so it may well be best to try to inform them of the outcome at the end of the interviewing session, as normally occurs in the education sector.

Carrying out this careful, planned and prepared approach to recruit-ment interviewing and devising suitable practical tests should result in recruiting 'right' persons from amongst the candidates who will do the job best and fit well into the department. It is a very expensive business if one gets it wrong, and so every effort should be made by health care managers to give recruitment, and the procedures attached to it, the priority that they need.

In practice, of course, there are few 'right' persons and often interview panels are faced with marginal decisions. If the panel has conducted its business well, it will have accumulated sufficient infor-mation from the selection process to reach a conclusion. This should be remembered by interviewers *during* the interview. They might ask themselves not 'what do I think about this candidate?' (which is itself a conclusion), but 'what have I learned about him/her that will enable me to make a fair decision and what more do I need to learn before the interview is over?'.

It is at the end stage, at the completion of all the interviews, that references can be considered. They may confirm or challenge recently-formed opinion and, where appropriate, particular points therein may need to be clarified by a telephone call to the referee. If decisions are highly marginal, it is not, by definition, worth splitting hairs in prolonged discussion, since either candidate could adequately fill thepost. After all consideration, a panel vote is the obvious way to resolve the matter.

Training

Once one has attracted and recruited the right calibre of staff, thentraining them to become competent members of the department becomes the priority. Training is provided to give new staff the basic skills they need for the jobs they will be expected to do, to improve performance and to provide new skills. The objectives of training are to produce skilled workers serving an efficient, well-run organization. This will, in turn, help to ensure a stable, loyal workforce and reduce or even remove costly labour turnover. The whole recruitment and training process is an expensive and time-consuming one, both for the staff involved and the employing authority. This is a further reason for wishing to retain staff of the right quality. Where training for new employees is concerned, it is necessary to decide initially whether staff are to be recruited directly into a specific role or department, or whether they are to be provided with a

'Cook's tour' of the depart-ment's work, and then given some choice as to which area of work they would prefer to concentrate on, and specialize in.

Training may take place at three main locations and the balance between them will depend on the particular health care profession concerned. The first is within the specialist department itself, the second will be at induction courses organized at unit, district or regional level by personnel and training staff, and the third will be at specialist training schools, colleges or polytechnics. Most initial training will, therefore, be at both internal and external levels. On-the-job training will mainly take the form of 'sitting by Nellie', being shown what to do by an experienced member of staff step-by-step, linked to job rotation around the various sections and areas of work within the department.

Off-the-job training usually takes place at a college or training school, where, for some professions, the emphasis has moved in recent years from skills acquisition to education and the pursuit of qualifica-tions with academic status. For any training programme to be effective it must result in the learning both of new skills and abilities. Learning has been defined as 'a description of behavioural changes which result from experience'.

The most common learning experience is slow at the beginning, it speeds up and gets faster, a momentum which is dependent on the interest of the subject-matter and the skill of the trainer in putting what he/she is teaching across to the trainee, and then it tails off, either earlier or later, depending on disinterest or fatigue. The skill and ability of the trainer is, therefore, vital in any effective learning process, and any member of staff who will be involved in training should themselves be appropriately skilled as trainers. Concern for training should be one of the departmental manager's key roles but he/she may decide its profile is best created and maintained by having someone with good teaching skills specifically designated as a 'training officer, whose main role would be to organize and encourage training, and possibly also to take on a large measure of the basic skills training themselves. Three essential aspects are required for efficient, effective learning:

1. The training needs to be spaced so that breaks are provided in the learning process, with shorter rest periods at the beginning and longer ones at the end, in order to eliminate fatigue.
2. 'Balanced guidance' is required to give the trainees enough help so that they do not become over-anxious and lose confidence which will affect their learning ability; however, it is equally important not to give too much guidance as this will lead to over-reliance on the trainer and ineffectiveness when the trainee tries to do the job on his/her own in the real job situation.
3. There is the need for feedback of information to provide motiv-ation. Trainees should be given immediate feedback information about their standard of performance, in order to boost their confidence if they are giving good performance, and to eradicate errors rapidly if they are giving inadequate or poor performance.

Once staff have been trained in the basic skills of the job, then they need to be developed and given the skills necessary for promotion. There may be a certain dilemma for a manager who has some excellent members of staff whom he does not want to lose. If they have reached the top of their incremental scale, and there is no scope for awarding merit rises in the NHS, and if there are no internal opportunities for upgrading or promotion, they will probably start looking elsewhere for a senior post. A poor manager might selfishly think that restricting staff development may be the best means of keeping them and reducing their chances of gaining promotion elsewhere. However, such an attitude is only likely to create frustration and demotivation amongst such members of staff and would be very shortsighted, as a good health care manager should be looking to develop the overall skills of all his/ her subordinates for the good of the NHS as a whole. Thus, all health care managers should be concerned with staff development which will often take the form of management training, as it is these skills which are most often required as staff move up the hierarchy in the various health care professions.

Retraining

This has become an important area in the last 20 years of rapid technological change, which has affected health care professionals both in the technology they use to carry out their work, and in the computing systems which are increasingly used to maintain and update patient records, results and appointments systems. The increasing desire of female staff to return to work after having children, and the increasing unemployment in some areas of the British economy, has also meant that the importance of retraining and its related research work has come to the fore. Retraining can be something that people either undertake voluntar-ily or are forced to do when they are relatively young—under 40 However, the importance of the topic really relates to people over 40 who, as they age, suffer from two major problems, the slowing of sensorimotor activities and the impairment of short-term memory. Research work by K.F.H. Murrell and A.T. Welford has identified these two major problems, and Welford lays the blame for poor performance in retraining by older workers on four factors:

1. Slowness in comprehension, which causes essential points to be missed in lectures and demonstrations.
2. Attempts to teach too much at once and thus overloading the short-term memory.
3. The fact that once wrong impressions are formed they are relatively difficult for older people to modify.
4. The difficulty which compounds these which is that middle- and old-aged people try to learn too fast.

Both Welford and Murrell feel, therefore, that special training methods should be developed for older people, particularly since, as workers, they often have a great many advantages over younger workers in terms of quality of performance, steadiness, reduced ab-sence, responsibility and the likelihood that they will be less involved in costly labour turnover. The problems of retraining older workers, and solutions to them, have been researched mainly by the Belbins at the Industrial Training Research Unit at University College, London. Their findingshave been very wide-ranging and detailed, but amongst the most important are that:

1. The training programme needs to be designed to remove as much anxiety as possible as this is likely to affect learning ability adversely.
2. As far as possible the training officer needs to deal with trainees on an individual basis rather than trying to apply a blanket, standard training programme.
3. Incorrect learning needs to be eradicated from the training scheme as 'unlearning' is particularly difficult for older workers.
4. The need for a trainer who presents himself as a colleague, and not a supervisor, and for the trainer

to maintain contact with the trainees when they first enter a job on their own, to solve difficulties and problems.

5. Mature adults learn better with longer sessions as concentration improves with age.

The Belbins have devised their own general plan for adult retraining called 'Discovery Learning', which develops systems that allow adults to play some part in organizing their own learning, and in so doing gives recognition to a basic and perhaps primitive need, linked to the fact that an adult is not a dependent and so provision for his training must be made on non-dependency lines.

It aims to bridge the gap between the training organization's need for controlled progress, and the recognition of the adult's desire to maintain his sense of personal freedom and identity during learning. It builds on the successes of the correspondence course, Open University, and open learning styles of instruction and learning. The onus of these courses is placed on the drive, enthusiasm, self-organization and self-discipline of the trainee to learn and train himself, within a guided learning programme. Health-care managers should thus acquaint themselves with such ideas if they decide to employ, update and retrain older staff who often do have qualities which young trainees lack, in order to make sure the retraining process is as smooth and effective as possible and, in turn, to ensure that older recruits are as productive and as satisfied in their new jobs as possible.

Management Training

In order to provide management training, it is necessary to identify those jobs which require management skills—an essential part of job analysis. There is also a corresponding requirement to identify people with management potential.

This is effectively achieved by a system of regular performance appraisal which will focus not only on task-related ability and problem-solving initiative but, where appropriate, on potential management skills: the willingness and ability to plan, communicate, control, motivate, delegate and to take decisions. It has been argued that appraisal schemes should preferentially relate to one purpose only per interview and we will develop this consideration. In practice, however, management potential is likely to be evident whatever purpose is attributed to the appraisal and those showing promise can be developed by being given genuine 'acting-up' opportunities when they arise.

It is a regional, and perhaps a district, manpower planning objective to identify the numbers of junior and senior posts in each occupational group that are required to meet current and planned organizational commitments. Naturally, this will relate to staff recruitment and training requirements. In this way, manpower planning forms an integral function with that of the personnel department. If it is also linked into corporate appraisal systems there then may be identified a pool of workers on which to base succession, contingency and recruit-ment policy and plans.

Identified 'high-flyers' may undergo further selection to differentiate their potential abilities. This could make use of the Assessment Centre facility where groups of trainees are put through a variety of observed management exercises and problem-solving situations. Evaluation studies of the Assessment Centre have differed in their findings,and we are unaware of any general use of this method of selection for management training within the NHS at this time.

Over the past 10 years or so, many health workers who hold, or aspire to, senior appointments have embarked on management courses leading to recognized qualifications.

Indeed some paramedical pro-fessions, the MLSOs and the radiographers, award their own qualifi-cations, as we have described in the Appendix. Other routes to a management qualification are the postgraduate Diploma in Management Studies, DMS, of which there is at least one course specifically designed for NHS employees,* and a variety of Masters courses concerned with management, business administration and other more specific topics relevant to particular aspects of man-agement.

In general, these courses are designed more to impart knowledge, to expose students to new concepts, to increase cognitive awareness of management issues and, *de facto,* to change attitudes than they are to develop requisite skills. That there is an important place for academic management courses and qualifications we would in no way deny. It is appropriate that those with potential or who are performing well with managerial responsibilities should be encouraged to attend appropriate courses and to obtain qualifications. Moreover, it is important to support participation in management training, both by encouragement and by financial assistance, and to recognize the qualifications gained in salary scale increments and conditions of service. To believe that knowledge of management issues is 'caught' rather than 'taught' is to discount the value of the concepts of management. Such knowledge is not necessarily conferred *inter alia* with that gained by the study of any other academic discipline, medical or otherwise, but depends upon a combination of awareness and opportunity, gained irrespective of occupational grouping and of which there may well be indication during the formal appraisal process.

Training for management, as opposed to management education, has traditionally taken the form of the 'training course' with, or more usually without, certification as an end product. Such courses are held centrally either at district or region and take employees away from their working situation in order to concentrate on an intensive pro-gramme of training. There is a tendency for some participants to view their mere attendance on these courses as a means to an end—a further substitute for their indifferent managerial performance on the job. In the changing culture of the NHS, they are likely to be disappointed. However, there is a need to examine why this should be so and to look at the weakness of the 'training course' approach and to identify some possible improvements.

One problem of the training course approach lies in the selection process; who is to attend? Departmental heads may be out of sympathy with the concept of management training and refuse to release staff to attend. This reaction is not as unlikely as it may at first appear. In a report to the Manpower Services Commission and the National Economic Development Office, Coopers and Lybrand Associates stated that training was:

> '... rarely seen as an investment but either as an overhead which would be cut when profits are under pressure or as something forced on the company as a reaction to other developments.'

The Report concluded that:

> 'If Britain's performance on training is to be improved—as we believe it must—this can only be achieved by a major change in employer attitudes to training; in turn, this will require changes in the environment in which they (employers) make their decisions.'

Alternatively, it is sometimes found that all staff, irrespective of inclination or ability, are nominated for management training due to the head of department's inability or unwillingness to be selective; to regard everyone as being entitled to their 'turn' of whatever good things are on offer or just to indulge in the short term redeployment of the poor performer in the hope that something of value will rub off.

Training courses vary from those aimed at first-line, middle and top management, frequently wide-ranging in content and often prescrip-tive in nature, to those designed to address specific functions or topics such as interviewing, appraisal, disciplinary and grievance procedures, computers, budgetary control and so on.

A successful course will enlighten many participants, give them fresh knowledge and insight and fire them with enthusiasm. However, when returning to their usual working environment, they are largely on their own facing the same historically entrenched problems that they had learned to abhor on the management course. Without strong and congruent support from the head of department and others, the implementation of change, be it of system or of attitude, is very unlikely to occur. Eventually peer group pressure to continue in the same old way as before takes its toll and the tangible benefit of the course is lost.

This is another problem of the 'training course' approach and is sometimes referred to as the transfer problem. In the 1960s and 70s it became the vogue to run experiential group training known as Encounter Groups, T-groups or simply Sensitivity Training. These are non-prescriptive, aim to be non-judgemental in nature and are relatively unstructured. Briefly, the aim of such groups is to help each member to identify and then publicly disclose those deep-seated problems that are inhibiting his/herhandling of social relationships and, therefore, of performance as a manager. Naturally, for such disclosures to occur, an atmosphere of complete trust is mandatory. This fragile concept was difficult to achieve and maintain particularly if participants were critical of each other. Without sensitive and experienced leadership ('strong' leader-ship was considered counterproductive) the group would either disinte-grate or degrade to a process of ritualization and playing safe.

We recall that initially there was enthusiasm for T-group training, some regarding it as a panacea for the solution of interpersonal problems at work. Clearly this approach does not suit everyone, although whether a worker is forced to attend such a course, is advised or self-selects may not be as important as other factors such as participant personality predispositions, perceived trainer style, the group training programme and individual participation. However, as with conventional courses, transfer problems have been found with T-groups.

The effect of these can be measured by questioning partici-pants and their working colleagues who have not undergone this training, at various intervals after the course to see to what extent training-induced behavioural change has been maintained. Apart from these considerations, there have been reports of psychological casualties during T-group work and some doubts cast on the applicabi-lity of this type of training for different personality types. References to these and other problems are given by Cooper and Bowles. On its own, then, the 'training course' approach is inadequate to meet the needs for which it was conceived, namely, to be the engine for organizational change. What is required to complement the formal (academic) management course is an approach which seeks to identify the changes and developments required, and the unresolved problems encountered, at a specific time within an organization. This will ensure that organizational and departmental aims, which are identified in the corporate plan, are subject to discussion with the 'trainer', the trainee, his head of department and others. In this way, specific training needs are identified and the relevance of training is perceived by the trainee and his colleagues and becomes *his or her* work-related project. As White asserts, 'it is the question of ownership that determines whether learning is translated into changes in behaviour at work and which is the fatal flaw in many off-the-job block management courses'.

This 'problem-oriented' approach to management and other train-ing is a new departure for training officers and means that, inevitably, their traditional role must change from that of giving the training to one of training consultant if they are to succeed. White argues elsewhere for training officers to concentrate much harder on diagnosis (of organizational problems) and evaluation (of the impact of training upon needs) rather than actually to conduct formal training which could in fact be 'contracted out' as he says 'formally or informally, within or beyond the district'. In the same journal Phillips and Tamplin describe a pilot project which identified the actual training needs of a mixed group of NHS staff. Individual trainees, their managers and departmental objectives were consulted and the findings analysed. The result was that 'different units and departments adopted a wide variety of approaches all of them relating to specific service needs'. Phillips and Tamplin report that 'individual learning require-ments are also being dealt with in the context of departmental objectives. We have noted a marked move away from putting on courses'. In this+ way, they believe, training is not seen as an optional extra but as an activity integral with achieving organizational objec-tives—an investment rather than a cost.

This approach may frequently mean that the training officer would be required to 'shop around' for suitable training facilities which might take the form of, for example, a short course, a Distance Learning package or specific counselling requirements. From a practical point of view funding for such training might be provided from the 'user' budget rather than centrally. Such an arrangement is compatible with the principle of management budgeting and would certainly focus the budget holder's attention on outcomes. A training 'consultant' is required to be thoroughly familiar with the district plan and to agree a strategy for achieving individual and departmental performance. Hul-lah emphasizes the need to follow up trainees to ensure continued support and encouragement and to establish that the whole operation has achieved the desired changes. She also believes that evaluation should place less emphasis on measures of declared client satisfaction and rather more on discovering if the required changes have occurred in the workplace.

Increasingly, the role of the training officer is seen to be merging with that of organizational development consultant. Briefly, this means that he is required to provide training to improve an organization's capacity for change by working with individuals, groups and departments. It is from this that he receives direction for his efforts and selects appropriate means to meet his clients needs. While reviewing management education, training and development in the NHS, the NHS Training Authority has called for:

- maximum participation by the individual in selecting and specify-ing the approach to be applied in his or her case
- the providers of development opportunities being explicit about their objectives
- individuals contributing their own values and experiences and not just acting as sponges of material fed to them

— a learning design relevant to the real issues being brought to the programme.

The report also considers that 'didactic teaching of academic sub-jects is not likely to change managerial behaviour'. This does not imply, we trust, that all academic students do not want or need to change their behaviour, merely that such courses offer them little help in doing so. Clearly the distinction is one between education and training. Until now the latter has been modelled on the former rather than making use of academic work to illustrate and explain.

LACK OF FEEDBACK

The final problem that must be dealt with arises in situations where information flows only in one direction. The quality control flow chart should be carefully reviewed to identify persons or committees who perform quality control tasks but who do not receive feedback on the effectiveness of their performance. A one-way information flow is bad management practice, and it also presents severe quality control problems. It means that the control loop is broken, making it impossible for the actors in the loop to evaluate the effectiveness of their behavior. A one-way flow of information calls the effectiveness of the entire quality control programme into question. Verification of the input is a critical management control function. A one-way information flow means that all the analysis subsequently performed on the input is of questionable value because the person generating the input cannot verify that person's work. The problem of one-way information flows should be handled by scheduling periodic group evaluation sessions. During the sessions, all the person involved in the control loop should meet and discuss their work and pose any questions they have about the input they receive from each other. These group sessions should be supplemented by formal evaluations. A formal evaluation must be periodically performed to ensure that the data that are processed in the quality control loop meet the criteria discussed earlier in the study.

IMPROPERLY QUALIFIED PERSONNEL

Unqualified or improperly qualified individuals who make quality control decisions pose both legal and accreditation problems. In many cases, the JCAH specifies the required training of individuals who hold administrative positions (such as requiring the head of nursing to be a nurse). The law requires that licensed professionals who are practicing their profession be supervised by licensed professionals. An administrator cannot tell a pharmacist how to mix drugs or tell a physician how to treat a patient. The administrator can set guidelines for these functions only in consultation with appropriately licensed professionals. This means that all quality control protocols that specify the way professional judgment are made must be approved by the appropriate professional staff committees.

REFERENCES

Bates DW, Cullen DJ, Laird N, Petersen LA, Small SD, Servi D, et al. Incidence of adverse drug events and potential adverse drug events: Implications for prevention. *JAMA* 1995; 274:29-34.

Cullen DJ, Sweitzer BJ, Bates DW, Burdick E, Edmondson A, Leape LL. Preventable adverse drug events in hospitalized patients: a comparative study of intensive care and general care units. *Crit Care Med* 1997; 25:1289-1297.

Felkey BG, Barker KN. Technology and automation in pharmaceutical care. *J Am Pharm Assoc (Wash)* 1996; NS36:309-314.

Glanville J, Lefebvre C. Identifying systematic reviews: key resources. *ACP J Club* 2000; 132:A11-A12.

Gotzsche PC, Liberati A, Torri V, Rossetti L. Beware of surrogate outcome measures. *Int J Technol Assess Health Care* 1996; 12:238-246.

Guyatt GH, Tugwell PX, Feeny DH, Drummond MF, Haynes RB. The role of before-after studies of therapeutic impact in the evaluation of diagnostic technologies. *J Chronic Dis* 1986; 39:295-304.

Harris RP, Helfand M, Woolf SH, Lohr KN, Mulrow CD, Teutsch SM, et al. Current methods of the U.S. Preventive Services Task Force. A review of the process. *Am J Prev Med* 2001; 20:21-35.

4

Hospital Evaluation Management Services

DOCUMENTATION OF EVALUATION AND MANAGEMENT SERVICES

The importance of documentation continues to grow. Failure to document properly can lead to payment denials with Medicare and private payors. In some cases, failure to document properly can be construed as fraud and abuse, which can lead to civil and criminal penalties. In short, if you don't document it, Medicare doesn't believe you provided the service. If Medicare finds lack of documentation in a postpayment audit, physicians can be liable for paying significant sums back to Medicare. HCFA became even more aggressive with the documentation issue in 1997. Late that year, new guidelines for documentation of evaluation and management services were handed down. These guidelines were onerous and would have forced physicians to provide extraneous services. Organised medicine rebelled swiftly and strongly, and HCFA delayed implementation. By mid-1998, HCFA had worked with the American Medical Association to develop a new set of guidelines. Specialty societies provided comments, which spurred HCFA and the AMA to continue the refinement process. By mid-1999, it was clear that while HCFA still intended to implement new guidelines, it would be some time before this happened. The American College of Rheumatology is participating in this refinement process to make the concerns of rheumatologists known to the AMA and to HCFA. When the new guidelines are finalized, the ACR intends to develop a template to help rheumatologists follow the guidelines as simply and quickly as possible. Meanwhile, Medicare audits continue. HCFA has stated that auditors will abide by the 1997 guidelines (which were so onerous and difficult to meet) or the 1995 guidelines which are less specific. The auditors have been instructed to follow the guideline that seems to favour the physician on a case-by-case basis. One drawback of the 1995 guidelines is that there is more room for interpretation by the auditor.

Nevertheless, most physicians feel that these guidelines are better than the 1997 guidelines. While there is no rule that physicians must follow these documentation guidelines, it is important to remember that auditors will not hesitate to seek repayment for services they feel were not properly documented. Medicare carriers previously audited less than 2 percent of medical records.

These audits were based upon billing profiles rather than random samples. In other words, you would only be audited if you displayed a pattern of inappropriate billing practices. Currently, carriers are also performing random prepayment audits for particular procedure codes. If you are chosen for an audit, the record reviewers will be looking for the information necessary to support your billing practice based on the documentation guidelines described in this chapter.

This study reviews the documentation guidelines for the three key components of E/M services and for visits which consist predominately of counseling or coordination of care. The three key components—history, examination and medical decision making—appear in the descriptors for office and other outpatient services, hospital observation services, hospital inpatient services, consultations, emergency department services, nursing facility services, domiciliary care services and home services.

Documentation of History

The levels of E/M services are based on four types of history: *problem focused, expanded problem focused, detailed,* and *comprehensive*. Each type of history includes some or all of the following elements:

— Chief Complaint (CC)

— History of Present Illness (HPI)

— Review of Systems (ROS)

— Past, Family and/or Social History (PFSH)

The extent of history that is obtained and documented is dependent upon clinical judgments and the nature of the presenting problem(s). The CC, ROS and PFSH may be listed as separate elements of the history, or they may be included in the description of the history of the present illness. In addition, an ROS and/or a PFSH obtained during an earlier encounter does not need to be re-recorded if there is evidence that the physician reviewed and updated the previous information. The review and update may be documented by (1) describing any new ROS and/or PFSH information or noting there has been no change in the information; and (2) noting the date and location of the earlier ROS and/or PFSH. The ROS and/or PFSH may be recorded by ancillary staff or a form completed by the patient. To document that the physician reviewed the information, there must be a notation supplementing or confirming the information recorded by others. Finally, if the physician is unable to obtain a history form the patient or other source, the record should describe the patient's condition or other circumstance that precludes obtaining a history. *To qualify for a given type of history, all three elements in the following "Anatomy of a Code" chart must be met.*

Anatomy of a Code

The descriptors for the levels of E/M services recognize seven components which are used in defining the levels of E/M services: *history, examination, medical decision making, counseling, coordination of care, nature of presenting problem* and *time*. The first of these three components (history, examination and medical decision making), are the *key* components in selecting the level of E/M services. An exception to this rule is the case of visits which consist predominantly of counseling or coordination of care. For these services, *time* is the key factor to qualify for a particular level of E/M service.

Documentation of an Examination

The levels of E/M services are based on four types of examination that range from limited examinations of single body areas to general multisystem or complete single-organ system examinations: *problem focused, expanded problem focused, detailed* and *comprehensive*. The extent of examinations performed and documented is dependent upon clinical judgment and the nature of the presenting problem(s). Specific abnormal and relevant negative findings from the examination of the affected or symptomatic body area(s) or organ system(s) should be described. A brief statement or notation indicating "negative" or "normal" is sufficient to document normal findings related to unaffected area(s) or asymptomatic organ system(s). *The medical record for a general multisystem examination should include findings about eight or more of the 12 organ systems.*

Documentation of the Complexity of Medical Decision Making

The levels of E/M services recognize four types of medical decision making: *straightforward, low complexity, moderate complexity* and *high complexity*. Medical decision making refers to the complexity of establishing a diagnosis and/or selecting management options as measured by:

1. The number of possible diagnoses and/or the number of management options that must be considered
2. The amount and/or complexity of medical records, diagnostic tests and/or other information that must be obtained, reviewed and analysed
3. The risk of significant complications, morbidity and/or mortality, as well as comorbidities associated with the patient's representing problem(s), the diagnostic procedure(s) and/or the possible management options

To qualify for a given type of decision making, two of the three elements in the following "Anatomy of a Code" chart must either be met or exceeded.

Documentation of an Encounter Dominated by Counseling or Coordination of Care

In the care where counseling and/or coordination of care dominates (more than 50 percent) the physician/patient and/or family encounter (face-to-face time in the office or other outpatient setting or floor/unit time in the hospital or nursing facility), time is considered the key or controlling factor to qualify for a particular level of E/M service. If the physician elects to report the level of service based on counseling and/or coordination of care, the total length of time of the encounter (face-to-face or floor time, as appropriate) should be documented and the record should describe the counseling and/or activities to coordinate care.

EVALUATING HIV/AIDS PREVENTION AND CARE PROGRAMMES IS A NEVER-ENDING CHALLENGE, BUT RECOGNIZING ITS IMPORTANCE IN IMPROVING CURRENT INTERVENTIONS MAY HELP TO ENHANCE THE SUCCESS OF FUTURE INITIATIVES.

There are probably as many definitions of "programme evaluation" or "evaluation research" as there are programme evaluators. Our approach to evaluating HIV/AIDS prevention and care programmes is best captured by a description of evaluation provided by Michael Quinn Patton:

> "I use the term evaluation quite broadly to include any effort to increase human effectiveness through systematic data-based inquiry. When one examines and judges accomplishments and effectiveness, one is engaged in evaluation. When this examination of effectiveness is conducted systematically and empirically through careful data collection and thoughtful analysis, one is engaged in evaluation research.... Evaluation is applied research, or a type of "action science." This distinguishes evaluation research from basic academic research....The purpose of applied research and evaluation is to inform action, enhance decision-making, and apply knowledge to solve human and societal problems....Applied evaluative research is judged by its usefulness in making human actions and interventions more effective and by its practical utility to decision makers, policymakers and others who have a stake in efforts to improve the world."

Such an evaluation approach is utilisation-focused. This approach emphasizes the interests of key stakeholders and primary users of the information at all levels, for example the donor, the host country, and the implementing agencies.

It applies socio-epidemiological research to identify ways to improve the design and implementation of HIV/AIDS prevention and care programmes.

Basic Considerations

Several considerations underlie the decisionmaking process about HIV/AIDS programme evaluation. The selection of an appropriate evaluation concept for an AIDS prevention programme is crucial because it determines the guiding philosophy behind the actual evaluation process. A number of theorists and evaluation practitioners have proposed various conceptual approaches to evaluation. These approaches differ in their conception as to what evaluation is, what the relationship with the primary client and other stakeholders should be, who should be making the relevant value judgments regarding the programme, and the criteria for judging the evaluation process itself. The conceptual approach debate was, and is for the most part, a debate about the best ways to measure and interpret change. It has highlighted a series of methodological dimensions among which there are variations in emphasis. These dimensions focus attention on some of the options available for making decisions about methods. Today, for example, there is consensus that both quantitative and qualitative data are valued and recognized as legitimate for programme evaluation. In fact, these methods are by no means incompatible and should be used in combination.

Deciding what and how much data to gather in an evaluation involves difficult methodological decisions and trade-offs between the quality and utility of information. An evaluation approach that uses multiple data collection methods, both quantitative and qualitative, is more likely to address diverse evaluation needs than is a more limited approach. At the same time, research priorities must be sensitive to competing needs for resources in an environment in which the HIV/AIDS epidemic is growing rapidly and evaluation is sometimes considered a luxury. It is a major task of the evaluator to match research methods to the reality of particular evaluation questions and to the available resources. There is also a need for evaluation researchers to play an active role, not merely a consultative one, in making design decisions for programme assessments. Although a programme evaluator should be a neutral scientific observer, he or she can also mediate between different stakeholder groups, can enable others through a participatory evaluation approach, and can advocate for the dissemination of evaluation results within the larger arena of decisionmaking. Planning evaluation and data collection activities in a participatory fashion is essential for achieving the delicate balance between practical needs and methodological desirability. Key stakeholders should be included in the planning process and every effort should be made for effective use of limited resources. Ensuring active support and participation of key stakeholders who have an interest in the results obtained by various data collection systems is particularly important for programmes funded by external donors that use host country institutions for data collection activities. Data produced by these efforts will have a better chance to be timely and of acceptable quality. Whenever possible, participants, including implementing institutions, host-country collaborators and local representatives of donor agencies, should attempt to reach consensus regarding data needs.

A Comprehensive Evaluation Framework For Country Programmes

HIV/AIDS prevention and care programmes need to be evaluated at different phases of the programme cycle. A framework for comprehensive programme evaluation. All stages of evaluation have to be considered together to provide an overall picture of the programme because no single data collection approach can supply all the information necessary to improve programme performance or affect policy change. Multiple complementary evaluation approaches and multiple methodologies (qualitative and quantitative) have to be applied to address different evaluation needs.

Formative Evaluation

Formative evaluation should be conducted during the planning (or replanning) stage of a prevention and care programme to identify and resolve intervention and evaluation issues before the programme is widely implemented. This is the time when flexibility is greatest and programme sponsors are freer to make decisions about how to proceed. Formative evaluation explores the need for interventions, provides the information necessary to define realistic goals and objectives for the programme interventions, and helps programme planners make tentative decisions about effective, feasible intervention strategies and how to carry them out.

Formative evaluation can also be used as an exploratory tool as the project is being carried out to provide feedback to project managers to help them adjust programme objectives to changing situations. Formative evaluation research can identify unacceptable or ineffective intervention approaches, designs, and concepts. Because of the urgency of the HIV/AIDS problem, many prevention programmes have rushed to carry out interventions without preparing first by conducting thoughtful formative evaluation. The lack of this type of evaluation is particularly felt in community-based interventions designed to reduce sexual transmission of HIV. In many cases, interventions have been based on ideas developed outside of the context of the lives of the people to whom the interventions have been delivered. The literature on behavioural change interventions is full of examples of ideas that made perfect sense in the abstract but failed completely in the "real world," mainly because the ideas were unacceptable to the target audience or were not stated in ways that were relevant to the lives of those people. A fuller understanding of the issues might well have led planners to redesign the intervention to make it more appealing to the selected audience. Fortunately, this situation is changing because formative evaluation is now being applied more frequently in designing prevention programmes. Formative evaluations use a mix of research methods that can rapidly provide relevant information to programme designers. These methods include:

— reviews of existing information;
— focus group discussions;
— individual in-depth interviews;
— participant observations; and
— short quantitative surveys with structured questionnaires

The most frequently cited methodological criticism of formative evaluation is its lack of external validity or generalizability. Because the results of the evaluation derive from small-scale rapid assessment procedures and/or pilot studies, one cannot generalize from them to a larger population. Despite this limitation, formative evaluation research can usually identify unacceptable or ineffective intervention approaches, designs, and concepts. However, even with adequate formative evaluation at the programme planning stage, there is no guarantee that a prevention programme will be effective when finally implemented; it may not be implemented adequately enough to be effective.

Process Evaluation

Once activities are underway, there is a need to examine whether they are being carried out correctly, on time, and within budget. Process evaluation addresses such basic questions as,

> "To what extent are planned intervention activities actually realised?" and "What services are provided, to whom, when, how often, for how long, and in what context?" Both input (the basic resources required in terms of manpower, money, material, and time) and output (the immediate service improvement expressed as distributed commodities, trained staff, and service units delivered) are key elements of process evaluation. These questions are often answered in quantitative terms. Qualitative evidence of how and why a prevention programme works or fails to work is equally important in answering process evaluation questions. Process evaluation requires getting close to data, becoming intimately acquainted with the details of the programme, and observing not only anticipated effects but also unanticipated consequences. An understanding of the processes through which intervention activities achieve effects can help to explain the outcome of the intervention. Process evaluation, however, does not demonstrate whether interventions are effective.

Process evaluation can also play an important role in improving or modifying interventions by providing the information necessary to adjust delivery strategies or programme objectives in a changing epidemic. Process-oriented evaluation is carried out throughout the course of the programme implementation and should use different methodological approaches to assess service delivery, ranging from reviews of service records and regular reporting systems, key informant interviews, exit interviews of service users, direct observations by 'mystery clients' (for example, in sexually transmitted infection [STI] and voluntary counseling and testing [VCT] services) to quantitative population-based surveys to assess programme coverage and barriers to service use. Different qualitative and quantitative study designs that are complementary to one another provide together the most comprehensive information.

Effectiveness Evaluation: Assessing Outcome and Impact

Evaluating the effectiveness of AIDS prevention programmes will almost always require quantitative measurements. These measurements will assess the extent to which the objectives of the programme were achieved. Effectiveness evaluation is used to answer the questions, "What outcomes were observed?" "What do the outcomes mean?," and "Does the programme make a difference?" Taking into account the various implementation stages of HIV/AIDS prevention programmes and the fact that, over time, new age cohorts become sexually active, it is advisable to stratify effectiveness evaluation by short-term and intermediate programme effects (programme outcome) and long-term programme effects (programme impact). Changes in HIV/AIDS-related attitudes, the reduction of risk behaviours and adoption of protective behaviours, and changes in STI rates are considered to be the most appropriate short-term or intermediate (also called proximate) outcome measures for interventions designed to reduce sexual transmission of HIV. Long-term effects include impact on HIV/AIDS trends, sustainability issues, and improved societal response.

Outcome and impact evaluation is intimately connected with process evaluation. Process information can help the evaluator to understand how and why interventions have achieved their effects and, perhaps, what is actually making the difference. Examining outcome/impact indicators without assessing the process of programme implementation could lead to erroneous conclusions regarding the effectiveness of the intervention. Programme goals and objectives have to be carefully defined to allow the selection of appropriate outcome and impact measures to assess the effectiveness of an AIDS prevention programme. Effectiveness evaluation is generally based on indicators that provide quantitative value from which the outcome and impact of interventions can be measured. Because multiple interventions working synergistically together are most effective in producing behaviour change, surveys should not be typically designed to capture the effects of one single intervention. Rather, they should be designed to measure behavioural trends in population groups who are exposed to combined interventions. The evaluation of one intervention is usually conducted through rigorous and expensive controlled trials.

Cost-effectiveness Analysis

Cost-effectiveness analysis also measures programme effectiveness, but expands the analysis by adding a measure of programme cost per unit of effect (for example, per number of HIV infections averted). By comparing the costs and consequences of various interventions, cost analyses and cost effectiveness estimates can assist in priority setting, resource allocation decisions, and programme design.

The Attribution Dilemma: Are Observed Changes A Result Of Prevention Interventions?

The ultimate goal of any HIV prevention programme is to reduce the number of new infections. Programme evaluation is intrinsically complex, however, due to the temporal evolution of epidemics and our poor understanding of how different behaviours and epidemiologic factors influence epidemic patterns as they move from an epidemic phase to an endemic state. Several factors unrelated to intervention effects can contribute to the observed stabilisation or decreases in the prevalence or incidence of HIV in a given setting. They include:

- mortality, especially in mature epidemics;
- saturation effects in populations at high risk;
- behavioural change in response to the experience of HIV/AIDS among friends and relatives;
- differential migration patterns related to the epidemic; and
- sampling bias and/or errors in data collection and analysis.

Determining whether observed changes in HIV incidence and prevalence are a reflection of the natural history of the epidemic or due to intervention effects is a critical evaluation issue. This is particularly true when evaluating behaviour changes in the face of growing numbers of people with AIDS-related illnesses because there is evidence that secular trends toward risk reduction will occur. For example, having a friend or relative with HIV/AIDS may influence adolescents to delay the onset of sexual relations or motivate those with non-regular sex partners to use condoms. Human sexual behaviour is influenced and shaped by many factors and exposure to an HIV prevention programme is only one of them. The question of whether behaviour changes can be attributed to prevention programmes, especially in countries with advanced HIV epidemics, has created some friction between stakeholders and programme implementers at the field level. Their different perspectives on this issue also reflect fundamental differences regarding the criteria for judging the process of programme evaluation itself. From a public health perspective, it may not matter whether the observed changes are due to a particular intervention. What is most important is that sexual practices have become safer and HIV infection should subsequently decrease.

From the cost-effectiveness or policy perspective, however, it is important to determine what caused the observed changes in sexual behaviour. If the changes would have occurred without a particular intervention that was designed to contribute to the observed changes, the costs of the intervention could be considered as resources better spent on something more useful4. Prevention programmes are under growing pressure to estimate which approaches work best for specific target populations in different epidemiologic settings with a given level of inputs in order to allocate resources in a cost-effective manner. Effectiveness evaluation, therefore, is critical because it can answer a basic question, "Does the programme make a difference?" A vexing task of assessing programme effectiveness is to disentangle the attributable affects of a prevention programme from the gross outcome and impact observed. Such estimates can be made with varying degrees of plausibility, but not with certainty. A general principle applies here: The more rigorous the research design, the more convincing the resulting estimate6. A hierarchy of evidence based on the study design can be established that reflects the degree of certainty in concluding that a given proportion of the observed changes in behaviour is attributable to the intervention programme and is not the result of other factors.

A ranking of different study designs according to their decreasing strength of evidence. Non-experimental observational methods with no control groups have been routinely used in behavioural outcome evaluations. It is important to recognize, however, that a before-and-after evaluation design with no comparison groups may be useful for assessing a prevention program's proficiency in delivering services, but it is not a very convincing design to measure programme effectiveness. The inference of cause and effect from such a design is problematic because competing explanations for across-time behavioural changes cannot be ruled out.

In some situations, the evaluation could assess "exposure" to an intervention programme or a specific element, and determine the extent of the association of that exposure with the desired outcome. This method, however, can be limited in its utility by factors such as lack of association of services or products with the intervention and inaccurate reporting by respondents of their participation in the intervention. The interpretation of programme evaluation data should always be approached with caution. In most situations, the programme and evaluation process as a whole is not a rigorously controlled experimental trial. The ability of an evaluation to precisely determine the true extent of a program's effectiveness is often limited by time, resources, and the lack of a rigorous design.

Many factors can confuse or confound the results measured, and biases can be introduced by a range of factors inherent to the problem of HIV/AIDS, the available measurement options, and those conducting the evaluation. One of the most difficult questions to answer in any evaluation is that of attributing any measured effect to the programme being evaluated. Defining the web of interacting and overlapping influences is extremely difficult, and is one of the reasons why so many programmes have difficulty attributing results to their actions. At some point, we need to stop worrying about attribution in such settings and focus on monitoring the changes as they occur.

The Role of Triangulation

Triangulation can be achieved through using multiple data sources, different researchers, multiple perspectives to interpret a single set of data, or multiple methods applied to a single programme, problem, or issue. In the absence of rigorous controlled trials, data triangulation procedures must be applied to substantiate a link between interventions and observed behaviour changes. For example, process evaluation data on condom sales, the intensity of peer education, or the quality and coverage of media campaigns can be combined with an analysis of behavioural outcome data to provide an understanding of the process through which an intervention has achieved its effects. Results from behavioural surveys should be analysed together with findings from qualitative evaluation research that is carried out in sub-samples of surveyed target populations. Such research can include focus group discussions, key informant interviews, and rapid ethnographic studies. This type of analysis will allow a more appropriate interpretation of observed outcome data because they are the likely results of the aggregate effects of multiple interventions as well as environmental and personal factors.

Many of the areas that need to be measured to evaluate HIV/AIDS programmes are sensitive and very personal in nature, such as sexual behaviours or personal attitudes toward persons with HIV/AIDS. Validity and reliability are critical issues for sexual behaviour research because the behaviours cannot be directly observed. Self-reports of sexual behaviours in the absence of additional evidence are often considered invalid and unreliable by stakeholders for whom such data are sensitive and run against firmly held cultural norms. One of the best methods for promoting reliability and validity, therefore, is to triangulate behavioural data with all other available and relevant biological, behavioural, and process data to explain more comprehensively the context in which risk behaviours take place. Given the abundance of AIDS-related research conducted in many countries, secondary data are a source of material for triangulation. Multiple-method triangulation is probably the most common triangulation technique. Rapid ethnographic research, combining semistructured information gathering with mapping, participant observation, and in-depth interviews, is another possibility. Focus group discussions have been widely used, as have individual in-depth interviews or key informant interviews, to obtain stakeholders' (or other key individuals') opinions about target groups' behaviour.

Finally, it is important to realise that behaviour change interventions have to be in place for sufficient amounts of time and on a large enough scale to have an impact on personal behaviour, social norms in communities, and ultimately on the epidemic. The example of Thailand shows that a focused intervention strategy implemented on a national scale can result in substantial declines in HIV incidence and prevalence in targeted populations. It is also an example of applied triangulation of data: STI/HIV trends were systematically collected by sentinel surveillance systems, and behavioural surveillance data provided the necessary supplementary information to interpret the observed epidemiological trends. There is now growing consensus that country programmes need to monitor risk behaviour trends together with trends in HIV infection.

Choice of Indicators

One of the critical steps in designing and carrying out an evaluation of an HIV/AIDS programme, or any programme for that matter, is selecting appropriate indicators. This can be a fairly straightforward process if the objectives of the programme have been clearly stated and presented in terms that define quantity, quality, and time frame of a particular aspect of the programme. Even with well-defined objectives, however, the choice of indicators for the evaluation of many programmes requires careful thought and consideration of both theoretical and practical elements.

The following questions can be helpful in selecting indicators:

- Is the focus of the objective a parameter that can be measured accurately and reliably?
- Are there alternative measures that need to be considered?
- What resources (human and financial) does the indicator require?
- Are there areas for congruency, either in the content of the indicator or the means of gathering the data?
- Are there any additional measures that would help in interpreting the results of the primary objective?

Selecting indicators and setting targets is usually done during the process of programme planning and replanning, preferably in a participatory way with the implementing agency and key stakeholders. Setting targets and benchmarks should also include information from similar types of interventions, so that the targets set are realistic from the perspective of the target population, resource allocation, and intervention type. While the level of attainment to be measured by the indicator is not actually part of the indicator itself, it is a critical factor. The magnitude of the level to be measured affects the size of the sample of the population needed to estimate that level accurately. It may also help evaluators select additional or supplemental indicators that might assist in later interpretations of the results.

Ideally, indicators should be:

- Valid—They should measure the condition or event they are intended to measure.
- Reliable—They should produce the same results when used more than once to measure the same condition or event.
- Specific—They should measure only the condition or event they are intended to measure.
- Sensitive—They should reflect changes in the state of the condition or event under observation.
- Operational—It should be possible to measure or quantify them with developed and tested definitions and reference standards.
- Affordable—The costs of measuring the indicators also should be reasonable.
- Feasible—It should be possible to carry out the proposed data collection.

Validity is inherent in the actual content of the indicator and also depends on its potential for being measured. Reliability is inherent in the methodology used to measure the indicator and in the person using the methodology. Many familiar outcome indicators in HIV/AIDS prevention, such as measures of condom use, provide challenges to the evaluator with respect to validity and reliability.

Interpreting outcome indicators for behavioural interventions that promote safer sex is further complicated by the fact that risk behaviours are measured in relative terms. For example, percentage figures of condom use measure the proportion of sexual exposures that are considered to be safe. These may or may not reflect the absolute number of sex acts that place individuals at risk for exposure to sexual transmission. Ten percent condom use in HIV-associated sexual episodes is still "safer" than 75 percent condom use in 100 HIV-associated sex episodes (9 versus 25 unprotected HIV-associated sex acts, respectively). Therefore, in this example it also would be important to determine the frequency of condom use in absolute terms in a given risk situation. Behavioural surveys have begun to address this dilemma by collecting additional data on "always or consistent" condom use in the context of sexual episodes with non-regular partners. Possible indicators related to different levels of programme evaluation The advantage of relating indicators to specific evaluation levels is that it also helps to identify opportunities for triangulating data. For example, survey data on condom use can be compared with information on condom distribution and availability in a defined intervention area. Or, available data on incident STIs, such as gonorrhea, in the surveyed population could be correlated with the condom data.

In collaboration with national and international partners, the United Nations AIDS Programme and the World Health Organisation (UNAIDS/WHO) have developed a standard set of indicators for country programmes that will refine and expand the prevention indicators (PI) developed by WHO's former Global Programme on AIDS (GPA). Moreover, because HIV/AIDS/STI prevention and care programmes are affected by many factors, including political commitment, available resources, and the socio-cultural and economic context, a new approach is currently being developed to capture the overall effort of national HIV/AIDS programmes.

The AIDS Programme Effort Index (API) is a composite score comprised of the main components of an effective national response. The potential advantage of this instrument is that it may yield useful information on the above issues even in the absence of more rigorous monitoring and evaluation systems. Using the key informant assessment approach, it also allows an assessment of areas that are difficult to capture with more objectively measurable indicators (e.g., political support and commitment). However, major concerns have been expressed with regard to the subjectivity and reliability of the API approach. The score depends entirely on the choice of informants, and the informants are likely to change from year to year. Questions have also been raised about the utility of a single composite score in which improvements in some areas may be masked by deterioration in other areas.

Differentiating Evaluation Efforts

Because of the various constraints on time, available funds, and trained staff, programme managers and evaluation planners must balance what is ideal or preferred against what is feasible, useful, relevant, and essential when choosing how to evaluate a particular intervention or programme. A useful approach for differentiating evaluation efforts is to define them in three different dimensions: the individual project dimension, the country programme dimension, and the international dimension. Using this multi-dimensional approach (individual, country, and international project) to set priorities for the degree of rigor needed to evaluate programmes and projects may alleviate some of the tension that arises when universal, standardized evaluation practices conflict with the objectives of individual projects.

One can think of the individual project dimension as an area of service delivery that, in most cases, does not require a rigorous research design to judge its proficiency, unless it is piloting a new intervention or responding to an unanswered research question, such as would occur with a demonstration project. Individual projects carrying out standard intervention strategies that have already been shown to be effective in other similar settings should focus their evaluation activities on formative evaluation (when needed for project planing), process evaluation, and capacity building assessment. The number of projects in relation to the different levels of evaluation efforts and reflects the current situation in programme evaluation. The monitoring and evaluation "pipeline" illustrates that there is usually a reduced number of projects that actually warrant the evaluation of the effectiveness of their implemented prevention activities. Within the dimension of a country programme, several categories of evaluation should be emphasized—intervention outcomes, socioeconomic impact, and changes in societal norms.

The guiding principle here is that in a situation in which multiple donors are conducting multiple interventions with overlapping target groups, certain types of evaluation are not appropriate for the scope of an individual project, but rather, should be coordinated and conducted by country or regional programmes. Use of such an evaluation approach, especially in the area of behavioural surveys, not only saves money, but also makes sense in environments where the effects of individual projects from different donors cannot be sorted out anyway.

Country programme evaluation includes (but is not limited to) the analysis of behavioural trends in different population groups in conjunction with an analysis of HIV/ STI surveillance data; the evaluation of social marketing activities related to condoms, drugs, and services; STI case management; scoring the overall effort of the national programme (for example, through the AIDS Programme Effort Index); socioeconomic impact assessments; and epidemiological modeling of the country's epidemic.

Countries will have different programmes of evaluation activities, reflecting their different information needs, which are determined by the stage of their epidemic, as well as their political and social environment, existing capacity for research, and available financial resources.

Evaluation efforts on the international dimension may address still existing uncertainties about which set of prevention interventions works best, in which setting, for whom, and under what circumstances (emphasis on cost-effectiveness analysis). This type of evaluation, however, requires large-scale community-based controlled trials that are certainly beyond the scope of individual projects or even national programmes. Given the difficulties and high costs associated with directly measuring the impact of HIV prevention programmes through large-scale incidence studies, more emphasis has now been placed on developing other methods of assessing impacts, for example through modeling. HIV/AIDS prevention and care programme evaluation is applied socio-epidemiological research whose main purpose is to identify and solve practical problems and guide programme managers and planners in improving the design and implementation of prevention and care activities.

This perspective not only determines the role of programme evaluation but also how an evaluation should be conducted, including the choice of indicators and levels of efforts in a given setting. By applying different methods from several disciplines to many types of problems, programme evaluation is a comprehensive research approach committed to meeting the needs of stakeholder groups as well as the requirements of the scientific community. This Handbook is designed to assist programme evaluators in this critically important task. Although programme evaluation is context specific, a comprehensive framework as outlined in this chapter is helpful in defining the questions that are to be answered by the different types of evaluation during the programme cycle. We advocate for a utilisation-focused evaluation approach that emphasizes the interests of stakeholders as the primary intended information users. To achieve the delicate balance between practical needs and methodological desirability, it is therefore essential that programme evaluations are planned in a participatory fashion with key stakeholders.

Decisionmaking is a political process and programme evaluators can play a major role in this process when evaluation efforts are expected to provide information of policymaking significance and relevance. Although evaluation researchers should be neutral scientific observers, there is also a need for them to assume a more active role and, if necessary, mediate between stakeholders with different and sometimes conflicting interests, perspectives, and information needs. Given the limited resources in most developing countries, assessing the effectiveness of HIV prevention programmes will often depart from scientifically ideal designs. In the absence of more rigorous evaluation designs, we urge programme managers and evaluators to apply triangulation procedures using multiple complementary methods as well as different data sources. Such a triangulated analysis will provide information comprehensive enough to allow a plausible and valid interpretation of observed outcome data, such as changes in risk behaviours, because they are the likely results of the aggregate effects of multiple interventions as well as environmental and personal factors.

REFERENCES

Bordley WC, Chelminski A, Margolis PA, Kraus R, Szilagyi PG, Vann JJ. The effect of audit and feedback on immunization delivery: a systematic review. *Am J Prev Med* 2000; 18:343-50.

Folli HL, Poole RL, Benitz WE, Russo JC. Medication error prevention by clinical pharmacists in two children's hospitals. *Pediatrics* 1987;79:718-722.

Grimshaw JM, Russell IT. Effect of clinical guidelines on medical practice: a systematic review of rigorous evaluations. *Lancet* 1993; 342:1317-22.

Hatoum HT, Catizone C, Hutchinson RA, Purohit A. An eleven-year review of the pharmacy literature: documentation of the value and acceptance of clinical pharmacy. *Drug Intell Clin Pharm* 1986;20:33-48.

Jenkins MH, Bond CA. The impact of clinical pharmacists on psychiatric patients. *Pharmacotherapy* 1996;16:708-714.

Ried LD, McKenna DA, Horn JR. Meta-analysis of research on the effect of clinical pharmacokinetics services on therapeutic drug monitoring. *Am J Hosp Pharm* 1989;46:945-951.

Schumock GT, Meek PD, Ploetz PA, Vermeulen LC. Economic evaluations of clinical pharmacy services-1988-1995. The Publications Committee of the American College of Clinical Pharmacy. *Pharmacotherapy* 1996;16:1188-1208.

5

Hospital Systems and Project Implementation

THE EVOLVING STATE ROLE IN THE IMPLEMENTATION OF THE RURAL HOSPITAL FLEXIBILITY PROGRAM

As indicated throughout this report, the pace of implementation in the Rural Hospital Flexibility Programme (Flex Programme) has increased dramatically in the second year. The number of hospitals that have converted to Critical Access Hospital (CAH) status has more than doubled. As important as these conversions are as indicators of programme success, there are critical, collateral activities—many of them undertaken by the states—that are also useful gauges of implementation success and, to a limited extent, of programme impact. The states' roles in the Flex Programme have been growing and evolving, from rural health plan development and implementation to providing funding and technical assistance for hospitals and communities to build and/or strengthen their rural health networks. In this second year, the Flex Programme Tracking Team conducted site visits in an additional eight states (plus a ninth state selected for an emergency medical service [EMS] visit). We also tracked continuing developments in the 12 states that were visited last year. Each of the state-level site visits was conducted by a team from one of the five collaborating rural research centers using a common, semi-structured site visit protocol. This protocol focused on most of the same issues covered in our first year site visits, but included additional items related to special studies that centers were conducting in this second year. Each site visit team prepared site visit reports, which have been shared and discussed by the Tracking Team.

What implementation strategies and activities have the states pursued, and how have these changed from the first year?

What successes and challenges have the states had in implementing this program?

What factors contribute to successful state-level implementation?

What are the future opportunities for continued development and success in the Flex Program?

Year 02: State Implementation Activities

State-level implementation activities are changing in response to the evolving needs and circumstances of the Flex Programme. In the first year of implementation, most states were focused primarily on developing policies and procedures for programme implementation, communicating with hospitals and others about the programme, and assisting with early conversions. With most of their "systems" in place, and conversions proceeding smoothly, many states seem to be moving to the "second generation" of the Flex Programme. Increasingly, these states are shifting their attention and priorities to a set of longer-term issues, including:

— Honing state priorities for the program;

— Focusing on longer-term rural hospital and health

systems performance issues by targeting technical assistance in areas such as strategic planning and quality improvement; and

— Beginning to focus on more difficult issues such as lasting structural improvement to rural EMS systems and the capital needs cf rural hospitals.

This evolution of state implementation activities is not surprising — we would expect this with the maturation of any programme like this one. What is especially important about the experience of these states, however, is that it may indicate the future directions of the Flex Programme. As such, this section summarizes the trends in state implementation activities and experiences that we have seen in this second year and examines the lessons that they might have for future Flex Programme priorities.

Conversion Activities

In each of the states we visited in the second year, the state office of rural health, state hospital association, state health facilities licensure and survey agency, and other organisations involved in CAH conversion activities had achieved a "steady state." That is, they had generally identified and worked out whatever problems they had encountered in the early phase of Flex Programme implementation. With the conversion mechanics established, states continue to spend the bulk of their time and resources conducting a set of core conversion-related activities, including:

Coalition-Building: Building and sustaining a coalition of hospitals and other organisations involved in and/or supportive of the Flex Programme has been central to the success of Flex Programme implementation in many of the states we have visited. States have developed and are supporting both formal and informal coalitions of interested stakeholders. Most states have sponsored annual or semi-annual meetings/conferences with CAHs, hospitals considering conversion, consultants and others involved in the Flex Programme. These meetings have become large events in many states involving a wide variety of participants including hospital staff and trustees, community agency representatives, state and county officials, hospital and other association representatives, elected local and state officials, EMS and licensure agency staff, and peer review organisations (PROs), among others. Participants we spoke with were uniformly enthusiastic and positive in their assessment that these meetings have had an important educational, technical assistance, and networking value.

Communication with Hospitals Recently Converted or Considering Conversion: The states we visited are all actively communicating with hospitals that had recently converted to CAH status and those considering conversion. Through these communications, the state implementing organisations are providing assistance on issues that the hospitals are encountering. They are also providing a means for the states to identify and monitor common issues across the experience of these hospitals.

Technical Assistance (TA) and Conversion Trouble-Shooting: The TA activities of the states we visited are focused primarily on: (1) helping hospitals assess the appropriateness of CAH conversion, (2) assisting with the conversion process, and (3) continuing to assist hospitals that have converted.

In addition to general consultation with hospitals considering conversion, states and their hospital association partners are providing support through the Flex Programme grants to assist hospitals to conduct financial feasibility analyses to determine whether conversion makes good financial sense. All of the states we visited are also providing various forms of TA to help hospitals successfully negotiate the conversion process. For example, virtually all states are assisting hospitals to prepare for the facility survey that precedes conversion. Many states are providing assistance to hospitals to develop and conduct their community needs assessments. Although states are required to demonstrate the development of only a single rural health network, virtually all the states we visited are actively encouraging the development of network relationships as a central component of the Flex Programme. Many states are using their Flex Programme grant funds to support hospital network development. In some cases, like North Carolina, the state office is providing assistance to CAHs to evaluate potential network partners and arrangements. The Flex Programme meetings and conferences that states sponsor are important vehicles for encouraging communications among potential network partners. Unlike the states' conversion assistance activities, the states' efforts to assist CAHs to identify community service, access or networking needs may encourage long-range planning beyond conversion. As CAHs stabilize their financial conditions, they face critical choices concerning the best means for rebuilding their market shares and re-positioning themselves in their local markets. To encourage and assist CAHs to move in this direction, several states, including Michigan, have been interested in developing TA assistance around strategic planning.

State Priorities and the Impact of Flex Programme Grants

The grant funds available through the Flex Programme to support hospital conversion and technical assistance activities continue to be vital to successful programme implementation. In Year 02, the federal Office of Rural Health Policy (FORHP) awarded $23.5 million in grants to the states. In most cases, state grant awards increased over amounts awarded in Year 01. In keeping with the changing focus of the states' TA activities, there has been a corresponding evolution in the states' priorities for the use of their grant funds. Whereas most of the grant funds in Year 01 were used to support hospital conversion activities, some states have begun to target the use of their grants to a wider range of state priorities for the Flex Programme. In some cases, these represent new priorities. In Michigan, for example, the state has introduced a priority for broad-based community health and social service agency involvement into their networking priorities for CAHs. This broader focus aligns Flex Programme objectives with existing state community health development initiatives. Other states, including Arkansas, have targeted the development of quality assurance/improvement activities. Consistent with last year's findings, however, the majority of states have used their grant funds to support:

- State activities associated with rural health planning activities;
- The CAH designation and conversion process at the state level (including survey and technical assistance functions);
- Hospital-level conversion activities such as community needs analyses and financial feasibility studies;
- EMS improvement activities;
- Quality assurance/quality improvement initiatives; and
- Rural health network development.

The majority of states we visited have targeted most of their grant funding either directly or indirectly to hospitals to support community studies, financial feasibility analyses, network development, and other activities associated with hospital conversions. States have also used their Flex grants to enhance their technical assistance capacity by hiring additional state staff or consultants. For example, Wisconsin has pooled some of its Flex grant funding to develop shared consulting contracts in five areas, including financial analysis, community needs assessment, telehealth development, staff development, and EMS assessment. The Center for Rural Health in Michigan, which has implementation responsibility for the Flex Programme, has used some of its Flex grant dollars to hire a physician recruiter to assist CAHs with their recruitment needs. The availability of Flex grant funds continues to be very useful in building hospital support for the Flex Programme and for the state offices of rural health. Grants have enabled the states to leverage interest, support, and commitment on the part of eligible hospitals, the hospital associations, and other stakeholders. Generally, states are limited in their regulatory leverage over hospitals through the licensure and survey process. Since these processes are not usually located within offices of rural health, the advent of the Flex grant funds holds the potential to strengthen the state offices' position as key players in the state.

There are significant variations in the scope of state implementation activities across the states. Many of our site visits have been to atypically larger states (e.g. North Carolina, Michigan, Texas) that have larger, well-established state office of rural health programmes. Many states, however, have small offices of rural health. Naturally, these smaller state offices have fewer staff and therefore more limited planning, technical assistance, and administrative capacity, and cannot undertake the same scope of implementation activity as the larger state office programmes. In general, the larger state office programmes have a greater capacity to anticipate and respond to the technical assistance needs of hospitals and communities, to engage in policy coordination activities, and to develop the policy and political influence needed to bring state government attention and resources to support the Flex Programme. In some cases, states have compensated for their small size and capacity by partnering with their state hospital association or other organisations to perform key implementation functions.

Both the federal government and the states have placed a priority on targeting as much Flex grant funding as possible to "on the ground" assistance to hospitals and communities. This priority has been reflected in the criteria used for determining the level of funding across the states. These priorities are understandable given the limited funding available under the Flex grant programme, and the interests of federal and state policy makers in helping hospitals move as quickly as possible toward conversion. Nevertheless, our site visits indicate that building state capacity to effectively implement the Flex Programme remains an important need in a number of states.

In some states, the limited staff and resources of the state office of rural health is inhibiting its ability to address some of the priority needs and activities identified in state rural health plans. Many of the rural health planning, community needs analysis, and technical assistance functions called for under the Flex Programme require specialized skills and resources that, by definition, are unlikely to all be found in a one-person state office of rural health. Unfortunately, the funding available under the Flex Programme in many states is not sufficient to enable the states to adequately fund grants to hospitals or other local entities (e.g., EMS provider groups) and use their Flex grants to add to their state office capacity to perform these functions. Adding to state administrative or programme staff is unlikely to be popular either federally or among the states.

Yet stronger state-level rural health policy and programme implementation staff and resources are needed if states are to effectively take on the full range of Flex Programme implementation and rural health plan management functions.

Lessons Learned and Policy Considerations

Many states, and especially those that have mastered the hospital conversion process, are looking beyond hospital conversions to identify new strategies for furthering the Flex Program's underlying goal of strengthening the rural health infrastructure. These states tend to view CAH conversions as a necessary but insufficient answer to the problems that rural communities face in sustaining (or developing) an appropriate rural health system. Among the key issues that these states are identifying are:

- — Sustaining or improving the quality of care provided in rural areas;
- — Addressing the capital needs of hospitals and other rural health providers;
- — Building an appropriate continuum of primary, specialty, acute and long term care services; and
- — Improving emergency medical care.

The agenda of needs and programme strategies are evolving; states appear to be developing a vision for the future of the Flex Programme. In doing so, it is important that they and others concerned with the Flex Programme consider the experience of the states to date and their implications for the future. Some of these lessons and their implications for the future of the Flex Programme are summarized in this last section.

Rural Health Planning and Policy Coordination

Rural Health Plans: In their second year Flex grant applications, many states indicated they would be updating their rural health plans. In the majority of states we visited, however, state officials noted that the process of updating their plans was a second or third-tier priority behind their conversion assistance and attention to other programme goals. The role and function of the required rural health plans required by the Flex Programme remain ambiguous and are not central to many states' programme implementation activities.

Designation Criteria: With the growing number of hospital conversions there is increasing federal attention being paid to the criteria that states are using to identify hospitals eligible for CAH conversion. In the first wave of site visits last year, we found that states were using a variety of criteria for designating CAHs and targeting grant funds and other technical assistance. Some states were being very inclusive in setting criteria while others were more narrowly targeting their CAH criteria and Flex grant funds. This pattern was evident in the Year 02 site visits as well.

Most states are using the provision in the federal regulations that allows for the state to designate "necessary" providers, thereby allowing hospitals that do not meet the 35 mile separation requirements to participate in the programme. This provision has been particularly important for states such as Nebraska where there are large numbers of small rural hospitals located relatively close to one another.

The typical strategy selected by states that adopt an inclusive approach to the programme is to broaden the eligibility criteria. This is most commonly accomplished by reducing the minimum allowable distance between rural hospitals from 35 miles as mandated in the federal regulations to as low as 15 (or fewer) miles and applying standards that allow hospitals to qualify as "necessary" community providers whose closure would present a threat to the health of the residents of the area in which they are located. These criteria generally involve some standard of demographic, health, or economic hardship. Typically, a hospital has to be located in a designated shortage area or in an area that has significant vulnerable, underserved populations as defined by the percentage of elderly and/or low income residents, the level of unemployment and/or uninsurance, and/or death rates from defined leading causes of death.

As discussed in this study, CAHs tend to be located in areas with limited health personnel and vulnerable populations, consistent with the states' designation criteria. As we reported last year, at least one state has tied its designation process to explicit expectations for CAHs. In North Carolina CAHs are expected to serve as safety net providers in caring for uninsured and other vulnerable patients. Although it is still early in the Flex Programme, more formal documentation of the extent to which CAHs are serving as safety net providers or are helping to build or sustain the local or regional rural health infrastructure could be very helpful in tracking programme success and in building or sustaining policy support for the Flex Programme. Developing the conceptual and methodological basis for doing such tracking is an important priority for the future of the Flex Programme.

Medicaid Policies: The involvement of state Medicaid programmes in the implementation of the Flex Programme has varied considerably over the first two years. In an increasing number of states we have visited, state offices of rural health and CAH hospital contacts report the growing importance of the Medicaid programme to CAHs. In particular, they have identified Medicaid payment for inpatient and outpatient services as a significant issue in implementing the Flex Programme. The importance of Medicaid payments to rural hospitals is likely to grow in the future as state Child Health Insurance Programmes and other Medicaid expansions are enacted and their enrollments mature.

In some states that have not moved to Medicaid cost-based reimbursement for CAHs, state offices of rural health are actively working with their Medicaid agencies and/or legislature to promote the adoption of cost-based reimbursement for CAHs. In other states, however, the state office has not even attempted to change current payment policies, either because they take a passive approach to policy development or because they know their efforts would be futile.

From our tracking work we know that fewer than half of the 47 states participating in the Flex Programme have established Medicaid policies to reimburse CAHs based on costs for outpatient and/or inpatient services. Some states, like Minnesota, however, have special Medicaid hospital payment methods that, although technically not cost-based, are at least as generous as cost-based payment.

In examining the role of the Medicaid programme, we were also interested in the impact that Medicaid managed care programmes might have had on CAHs, especially where those programmes (e.g. Michigan, Tennessee) require that CAHs accept capitated or discounted payments for services provided to Medicaid beneficiaries. The stories we heard were mixed. In Michigan, Medicaid managed care does not appear to have been a significant problem for CAHs. For example, where most hospitals are paid discounted rates by the handful of plans that offer a Medicaid product, one hospital administrator, although not enthusiastic about the rates he was being paid by the plan, was actually optimistic about the potential benefit that a greater volume of Medicaid business could have for his hospital. In contrast to this Michigan experience, we learned in one CAH in Tennessee that physician payment rates under TennCare had prompted physicians to leave the programme, resulting in the CAH having to cover the care for Medicaid beneficiaries unable to access physicians in the area.

In addition to whether Medicaid pays cost-based reimbursement, our site visit findings indicate that it is also important to consider the impact of other Medicaid programme features and policies on the Flex Programme. These features include, for example, Medicaid eligibility and benefits policies, payment policies affecting Rural Health Clinics, Federally-Qualified Health Centers and other rural "safety net" providers, disproportionate share policies, and Medicaid policies governing long term care payments, eligibility/patient assessment, and swing beds.

In West Virginia, for example, where CAHs are paid on a cost basis under Medicaid, we discovered the state's disproportionate share policies (DSH) have created a significant incentive for CAH conversion. Specifically, the state calculates most hospitals' DSH payments by summing their charity care and Medicaid "discounts." Most hospitals are entitled to 50 percent of this amount. CAHs, however, receive 100 percent of this amount, providing a significant incentive for hospitals to consider CAH conversion. This differential diminishes in subsequent years because of Medicaid cost reimbursement.

Minimum Data Set: Hospitals with swing beds are currently required by Medicare to complete the Minimum Data Set (MDS) assessment on all swing beds patients. In the second wave of site visits, this requirement was identified by state and hospital officials as costly, burdensome, and unnecessary given the nature of the swing bed programme. The American Hospital Association and others are actively working to change this policy.

Variations in State-Level Implementation and Building State Rural Health Development Capacity

As indicated above, we have observed significant variations in the resources available to state offices of rural health for the implementation of the Flex Programme. Some states, like Minnesota and North Carolina, have large rural health programmes with many staff, multiple programmes, and diverse sources of federal, states and foundation funding for rural health initiatives. Many other states, however, have fewer staff (some are one-person offices), are smaller, and therefore, offer fewer services and programmes.

As might be expected, these smaller offices face greater challenges in implementing the Flex Programme. With fewer staff, they have to rely on their partnerships with the state hospital association, other state agencies, or other organisations to provide assistance with the implementation of the programme.

These variations are associated with differences in the scope of Flex Programme implementation across the states. However, the size of the state and its rural health programme alone are not adequate for explaining the variations in implementation experience across the states. For example, as states like Montana demonstrate, political and policy leadership and advocacy on behalf of rural health are usually more important than size in determining the effectiveness of the state's rural health programmes.

In order to understand better the characteristics of

states and how they might be influencing the implementation of the Flex Programme, we have used our 20 state-level sites to create composite portraits of the states. For the sake of discussion, we see three categories of states:

— The "early adopters,"

— The "in process" states, and

— The "emerging" states.

We purposely use non-judgmental terms in labeling these categories because we are not interested in judging states. Our aim in characterizing the states in this way is to understand better how and why states differ in their approach to implementing the Flex Programme and in their commitment to and capacity for rural health development.

"Early Adopter" States: States in this group have responded quickly to the opportunities afforded by the Flex Programme in order to advance pre-existing state rural health priorities. As such, they have clear policy priorities that are reflected in their use of Flex grant funds, in their designation criteria, and in their implementation support and other activities. As the programme has evolved and conversion activities become more routine, states in this group have identified new needs and priorities and developed corresponding policy and programme initiatives. These states have moved quickly and effectively to develop coordinated policies and procedures for enabling hospitals to covert to CAH status. They have also marketed the programme widely to a broad range of rural health stakeholders, primarily rural hospitals and communities, and to policy makers. The states in this group have built a strong coalition that provides a base of political and policy support for rural health generally and the Flex Programme specifically. Other distinguishing characteristics of these states include the following:

— They have developed a critical mass of technical assistance, policy development, and demonstration or assistance staff, programmes and/or resources;

— The office of rural health has gained support from rural health constituencies;

— The state is involved in strong partnerships with other organisations concerned with rural health;

— There is strong and influential political and policy support for rural health in the legislature and/or governor's office; and

— The state has a history of policy interest and investment in rural health programmes (e.g. health personnel programmes, network development programmes, capital assistance programmes).

"In Process" States: The states in this group tend to be characterized by the ad hoc, grant-driven nature of their rural health programmes. They have sought and obtained available grant funds to support a variety of rural health initiatives, but have not yet achieved the degree of programme synergy that characterize states in the "early adopter" category. Most of the rural health funding in these states tends to be federal, with only limited state support. This situation reflects the more limited base of policy and political support for rural health in these states, compared with the "early adopter" states. This more limited base of support reflects the fact that these "in process" states do not have strong coalitions of stakeholders. Implementation of the Flex Programme in these states has focused primarily on hospital conversions, with more limited attention to rural health network development, community development, and other priorities embedded in the programme.

"Emerging" States: These states tend to be characterized by their dependence on federal grant support for all of their

rural health activities. In fact, without such funding, it is unlikely that they would support an office of rural health. This reflects the limited policy and political support for rural health in the state. Because of their dependence on federal grant funding, the state offices of rural health in these states tend to be small, with limited staff and resources for carrying out their functions. If these states have stakeholder coalitions, they tend to be weaker than in other states and to have a limited policy impact. Implementation of the Flex Programme in many of these states has been slow, with few CAH conversions. Other state office activities and functions, such as technical assistance, have also been limited.

State political cultures affect the degree of state direction and leadership that is possible or desirable in any particular state. Nevertheless, it is clear that strong state leadership and capacity make a big difference in rural health development. The states that we have described as "early adopter" states have generally been more successful in implementing the Flex Programme than states with a more limited commitment to and capacity for rural health development.

What does "state capacity" mean in the context of the Flex Program? Most importantly, it means having strong leadership that can catalyze interest and support among stakeholders for an agenda for Flex Programme implementation. This leadership can come in the form of a strong state office of rural health director, or through a coalition of rural health stakeholders who, together, are able to articulate a clear and compelling agenda. Beyond having a clear agenda and the leadership behind that agenda, it is also critical for states to have a critical mass of resources needed to move that agenda forward. Here we see a dilemma that many states face in the Flex Program: how much of the resources of the Flex Programme should be used to support state-level planning and technical assistance functions and how much should be directed to local hospitals and communities for community health improvement initiatives? The answer to this dilemma, of course, is that both are needed. In many states, the current funding levels in the Flex Programme are not sufficient to achieve balanced investments in both of these areas. Although we are only two years into the current programme, we are already beginning to see an important evolution of state priorities and activities. States that have mastered the hospital conversion process are turning greater attention to the more ambitious "second generation" goals of the Flex Programme of promoting and building sustainable rural community health systems. The experiences of these states deserve careful consideration as federal and state policymakers consider priorities for the future of the Flex Programme.

Programme Focus: Hospitals and Communities

As state priorities evolve toward greater attention to community rural health improvement, the potential tension between the hospital focus of the Flex Programme and broader community health system development may become more significant. The prevailing vision behind the current Flex Programme is that through CAH conversion, small rural hospitals will shift their orientation and service base to become community health service institutions. While there are clear examples of where this has happened, there are also many examples where hospitals have been exclusively focused on short-term survival needs and, understandably, have paid little attention to the community health system development priorities in the programme. We are only two years into the Flex Programme. Hence, more hospitals may turn their attention to these longer-term rural health systems development priorities if and when their financial conditions stabilize. As the Flex Programme evolves, it is important that financial and other incentives and support resources be more explicitly targeted to broaden the rural health development priorities, if hospitals and other community health care providers are to be encouraged to move beyond short-term hospital survival concerns to address the broader community health needs of their communities and regions.

Aligning Federal and State Goals and Programme Strategies

In our report last year, we noted that the majority of states we visited were measuring success in the Flex Programme by the number of CAH conversions. This was to be expected given the press of managing the first wave of conversions in most states. We questioned, however, whether and to what degree the goals beyond hospital conversion, including rural health network and infrastructure development, would receive the same attention as the conversion process. As we have noted in this study, an answer to this question is beginning to emerge. States have begun to shift their attention to new priorities and strategies beyond promoting and supporting hospital conversions. These priorities were variously described as "helping hospitals and community health systems become sustainable," "improving the performance (or quality) of rural hospitals and other providers," and "addressing rural community health needs." However these priorities are described, they speak to the underlying goals in the Flex Programme of helping to stabilize and build an appropriate and sustainable rural health system. The "early adopter" states are pioneering the vision and strategies for defining what constitutes a "sustainable, appropriate rural health system." The lessons of these states can and should be used to set the future goals, direction, and strategies of the Flex Programme.

The incentives and resources of the Flex Programme could be clarified and strengthened to help states and communities move toward this larger vision for rural health improvement. As a predominately hospital-focused initiative, the program's incentives for broader community-based rural health system development are limited. Although states and hospitals are undertaking a variety of interesting and important rural health improvement initiatives using Flex grant funding, these tend to be small and localized.

States (and their community and rural health provider partners) will certainly need greater resources to address their rural health development needs more systematically or comprehensively. Most importantly, however, those resources need to be tied to a broader set of rural health development goals. Those goals might focus on strengthening the rural health safety net for vulnerable populations, enhancing appropriate service capacity in rural communities, and/or improving the performance of rural health systems. Goals such as these would dovetail very nicely with the criteria many states are using to designate CAHs as essential hospitals. In addition, as suggested by the example of North Carolina, programme strategies such as technical assistance and Flex grants could be targeted more explicitly to activities and initiatives that aim to help hospitals, other rural health providers, and rural communities achieve these goals.

HOSPITAL CONVERSION PROCESSES

Rural hospitals continue to play a major role in providing health care services to the nation's 54 million rural residents. However, over the last few decades hundreds of these hospitals have been forced to close their doors. The continued struggle of rural hospitals to meet local health care needs has a multitude of causes, including technological, demographic, economic and policy changes, as well as decreasing capital reserves, aging physical plants, and rising numbers of the uninsured and underinsured. Small hospitals are at particular risk because of their heavy dependence on Medicare reimbursement to cover operating costs.

This study provides observations about the conversion experiences of hospitals participating in the Flex Programme. Data for the chapter were drawn from the telephone survey of 217 CAH administrators, the sixteen CAH site visits conducted during the second year of our project and information collected by the University of North Carolina (UNC) on hospital characteristics and participation in the Flex Programme. Observations of the first two years of the Flex Programme suggest that the hospital conversion and network development experiences of programme participants have accelerated due to pressures such as aging physical plants, lack of capital, and lagging technological infrastructure. It is as if CAH conversions have been influenced by a compelling need to "do it now" and "do it quick" to avert closure. It is natural and tempting to search for programme impact as soon as conversions occur. However, given the market and industry conditions that have faced the rural areas represented, care should be exercised in drawing conclusions at this early stage.

Hospital Conversion Experiences

Lessons Learned

Hospitals, states, and stakeholders participating in the Flex Programme have reported a number of lessons learned that they felt should be shared through the Tracking Project. The information and recommendations they provided were consistent with the Year 01 findings. Nine key lessons have been sorted into three areas: 1) the strategic frame of conversion to CAH; 2) conversion support for success; and 3) conversion trip points.

(1) Strategic Frame

It is still too soon to be sure what aspects of hospital characteristics or programme relationships may have the most influence on making successful conversions and, more importantly, maintaining successful operations after conversion. The key theme for the four lessons below is that a hospital administrator runs a risk of failure if it is assumed that any single provision of the programme is sufficient to stave off closure. Success depends upon the ability of managers to engage in ongoing efforts to assess, evaluate and integrate their efforts within a context that accommodates the immediate needs of their facility relative to existing market conditions, and also considers the potential implication of such actions for other key players in their market area.

— Cost-based reimbursement should not be the only reason to convert.

— Don't wait to convert; if you are sure of the facts—act on them.

— Find out what other hospitals have experienced in their conversion process.

— Working with the community can be difficult but is important for a successful conversion.

(a) Cost-Based Reimbursement: The fact that most of the hospitals participating in the Flex Programme are in poor fiscal condition is probably the single most important factor behind respondent reports that financial need was a key reason to convert. Three-quarters of the 164 administrators providing pre-conversion annual income figures in the survey reported losses (averaging $200,000). However, many administrators recognized the danger of placing too much emphasis on reimbursement in the conversion decision.

CAH reimbursement under Medicare pays only "allowable costs" and obviously pays only for Medicare patients. A few survey respondents and administrators interviewed during the site visits related instances where colleagues had used financial opportunities (not necessarily Flex Programme opportunities) to make-up for cash shortfalls rather than using them to position their facility in a more adaptive and flexible operational mode. The former strategy postpones the inevitable by focusing on maintaining the status quo while the latter enables the organisation to better adapt to changing market demands by underwriting structural and operational change.

(b) Don't Wait to Convert—If You Are Sure of the Facts, Act on Them: Change is hard to embrace for most individuals and it is even more difficult for organisations because of the variety of interest groups and stakeholders involved. Given the poor financial position of many hospitals considering conversion to a CAH, it is possible to wait too long to make the conversion decision. A number of respondents emphasized the importance of acting prudently but promptly in the decision to convert. They recognized that good information was the key to making timely and effective decisions about organisational change, and emphasized the importance of good management and leadership.

While some participating hospitals have expanded existing services and added new ones, the larger facilities that are now becoming CAHs will face more difficult choices. Participation in the CAH programme may require these hospitals to reduce the size of their operations significantly (such as reducing inpatient capacity while increasing ambulatory capacity, or retraining and replacing staff resources). Administrators facing more significant operational changes may postpone conversion either because of the desire to re-analyse the data or because the decision is difficult or painful. Administrators who have faced such decisions have discussed the agonizing process of reducing their workforce (e.g., meeting "downsized" individuals or their relatives in the local park, bank, or grocery store). The smaller the community, the more difficult the human aspect can become. But this does not change the fact that if action is not taken, the hospital could lose its role as an employer altogether.

It is also not surprising that some administrators delay conversion decisions because they have hopes that their hospital will be saved by a last minute state legislative appropriation or low/no-interest loan (stories of such rescues have persisted since the Essential Access Community Hospital/Rural Primary Care Hospital [EACH/RPCH] Programme and, to a degree, continue today).

Administrators who have made the decision to convert recommend that conversion be scheduled for the beginning of the month. This is similar to a recommendation last year that conversion be scheduled for the end of the hospital's fiscal year to make it less expensive (i.e., avoiding multiple audits) and easier on the people involved. It is also advantageous, if feasible, not to be the first in the state to convert. Unfortunately, those hospitals seeking to convert are often in the worst financial condition. Those fortunate enough to become affiliated with network providers with a strong commitment to their partners and access to sufficient resources are able to negotiate the transition with far greater aplomb, and are better prepared to begin successful post-conversion operations. For example, a CAH that has a strong collaborative relationship with a larger hospital has better opportunities for obtaining bridge loans from local lenders or from the support hospital.

(c) Find Out What Other Hospitals Have Experienced:

A number of respondents strongly recommended consultations with administrators who have already gone through the process. "Networking with CAHs can be very helpful in sorting out issues." However, it is important to remember that each hospital's circumstances will be different and therefore subject to varying degrees of influence from community, physicians, nurses, state level staff, and others. One respondent made the important observation that it is more helpful to get advice from hospitals that converted later in a state program's history than earlier, when the learning curve was steeper. In other words, it helps to find out how things should work in order to foster similar conditions for your own hospital's conversion.

(d) Working with Communities Can Be Difficult, but It's Important: As with the information collected last year regarding the pros and cons of involving community representatives in the conversion process, there was a range of opinion among the respondents. Many pointed out that it was critical to obtain the needed support of the community. When looking at the choice of words used by administrators regarding the community, "community involvement" often was seen as a process of community members educating rather than sharing decision-making authority or inviting outside expertise.

Last year one of the hospital respondents made the statement that is was wise to "invite them (community representatives) to dinner but not into the kitchen." This year an administrator commenting on the need to educate the community about the circumstances of the conversion stated, "This is the decision, these are the reasons—we're not asking for permission." Such comments do not appear to reflect a defensive posture on the part of hospital administrators, but rather convey an attempt to maintain a balance between civic awareness and market realities.

Several administrators pointed to the important role of community outreach and involvement for post-conversion success (e.g., it is critical in terms of marketing the services that a hospital hopes to provide). One respondent noted that while community outreach requires a lot of work, it can be very important for building market share.

(2) Conversion Support for Success

Conversion to a CAH, while definable in discrete events and activities, is very much an evolving process. In order to navigate successfully through a maze of negotiations, agreements, transitions and re-organisation, a number of efforts must be in play simultaneously. Tracking and evaluating the cumulative impact of these multiple efforts requires a significant investment of time, energy and resources. Anything that contributes to a smoother and more open process facilitates oversight and coordination, as well as achievement of a successful outcome. Three recommendations for achieving a smoother and more open process include:

- Management teams should include individuals with strong financial skills.
- Work with the Medicare Fiscal Intermediary early in the process.
- Keep physicians and other staff informed.

(a) Management Teams Must Have Financial Skills: The process of conversion can be extremely complex in that its success depends upon very close attention to detail. Given the many financial implications of the conversion, the more that management "understands the ins and outs of cost-based reimbursement, the better they can make it work for their hospital." It also helps if the chief executive officer (CEO) has strong financial skills to develop services and manage costs. As one respondent indicated, "CAHs

have to manage their numbers and not be managed by the numbers." It is the CEO who usually represents the hospital's strategy before the board, the community, and other interested parties. Another respondent supporting this position noted that "without good management, CAH conversion is not going to save a hospital." Some of the administrators noted that management styles with demonstrated success in the private sector can be adapted to hospital operations to improve their efforts to monitor, plan and evaluate operations (particularly in terms of forecasting and assessing of potential operational strategies).

For example, it was mentioned that hospital managers are increasingly called upon to support initiatives that have economic implications for the community (e.g., as a condition of business relocation to the area, business might demand 24-hour emergency room coverage by board certified/ eligible physicians).

Situations like this will become ever more important as a hospital's status depends upon retaining good favour in the community in order to maintain local subsidies and credits. To improve their chances of survival, managers must be able to balance these opportunities to forge stronger links with their community.

(b) Work with the Medicare Fiscal Intermediary Early: The need to work closely with the Medicare Fiscal Intermediary (FI) continues to be a major suggestion from administrators who have converted to CAH status. Last year it was noted that a common problem for converted hospitals was the length of time between designation and the receipt of CAH-based reimbursement from Medicare. This continues to be an issue, albeit one that diminishes as the number of states and CAHs participating in the programme increases and learning curves level out. The

most important reason given for working with the FI early was the same this year: to "avoid a lag in payments and ensure that an appropriate interim rate is established."

(c) Keep Physicians and Other Staff Informed: The majority of the administrators site visited this year stressed the importance of "doing one's homework" and getting medical staff support early in the process. While some favoured education and information over involvement in the process, it is unclear whether this reflects their desire to retain authority over the process, or merely a recognition of the time and energy constraints of their medical staff. Respondents were clear about the need to make sure that the board, medical staff, and nursing staff understood the reasons for conversion and the implications of taking such action. While a few cautioned that one should not oversell the issue, most were clear that a common understanding needed to be established not only to answer questions but to facilitate the open dialogue so necessary for successful conversion.

(3) Conversion Trip Points

Last year three lessons were identified that were considered potential trip points for the conversion process: being confident in the financial feasibility study, focusing on the human as well as the organisational aspects of conversion, and questioning future funding promises and projections when making a conversion decision. This year's lessons share some overlap with those identified last year.

- Question your feasibility studies, particularly if conditions change.
- Be aware of the organisational culture prior to conversion.

(a) Question Your Feasibility Study: A large number of

respondents pointed out the importance of trusting the figures from financial feasibility studies. Clearly, these studies are critical to the conversion decision, and the more the management team understands the financial aspects of conversion, the greater the chance of making appropriate decisions. However, several respondents noted that it is important to remain aware of changes that can emerge after the analyses are completed. If this happens, several respondents pointed out the need to challenge the study before moving too far along in the process.

It is equally important to "look at the potential changes in hospital operations and decide if you are willing to change and if it is going to be worth it." The importance of being able to forecast the implications of organisational re-engineering can be vital. Given that more than two-fifths of the surveyed CAHs used internal personnel to perform their feasibility assessment, these tips take on particular relevance. Unless a hospital's situation is very straightforward, it is advisable to find someone with experience using cost report data to examine the feasibility of operational changes, and to assess the implications of conversion for external as well as internal operational relationships. It is also advisable to review all contracts and operations for possible savings as well as implications for changes following conversion.

(b) Be Aware of the Organisational Culture Prior to Conversion; It is easy to view conversion activities as mostly technical processes: crunching the numbers, gathering opinions, making decisions, and acting accordingly. However, as noted in last year's report, it is important to remain aware of the subtle human element in the process and the potential for interpretations and attributions that can alter the context surrounding decisions to convert. For example,

in one facility an existing management contract covering the hospital CEO and the director of nursing (DON) complicated conversion efforts because it increased the suspicion among staff that the change was being forced from the outside rather than internally. At another site, a historically high turnover rate among administrative staff led to a power vacuum filled by nursing staff. As the conversion proceeded and the nursing staff were not involved to the degree they considered appropriate, significant issues arose requiring negotiation before the process could successfully continue.

Reasons for Conversion

The CAH administrator survey asked respondents to identify up to two of the *most important* reasons for conversion. In some ways this question measures key threats facing the administrators prior to conversion. The open-ended responses were grouped into broad conceptual categories for analysis. Over one-half of the administrators identified financial distress or some action needed to avoid or forestall closure (52% payment and 6% survival-related). About a third of the administrators reported the primary motivation for conversion involved program-related or strategic issues, and the remainder cited community issues, state/federal health policy and regulations.

Payment Related: By far the vast majority of administrators cited concerns about finances, reimbursement and their hospital's bottom line as the most significant reason for conversion. The strong attention given to the financial need of these facilities is not surprising given the crisis mode under which many have been operating for years. However, several CAH administrators cautioned that it was critical to keep the financial crisis in perspective. If the financial crisis is the only focus, it can prevent administrators from recognizing other issues that underlie the larger financial problems. In other words, financial viability should be addressed from a balanced perspective that focuses on those factors that have contributed to the crisis, as well as those that may be projected to emerge as rural hospital markets continue to evolve. If a balanced approach is not adopted, the long-term survival of the hospital becomes problematic.

There were also administrators who reported that the development and organisation of new services was often a struggle requiring them to juggle the need for fiscal viability with the desire to meet community needs. Several noted that cost-based reimbursement under the Flex Programme opened up additional options (i.e., developing new services that are needed, or serving primarily Medicare recipients). A number of administrators pointed out that private sector management styles provided important lessons for operating their public sector facility. If they could not find effective strategies for stabilizing their financial viability it would become increasingly difficult, if not impossible, to address community health care needs.

Programme Related: Twenty-one percent of those surveyed listed program-related reasons as a key factor in the conversion of their hospital. For some, this response illustrated the ease of transition because they already fit the bill—"Didn't need to change a thing—We fit the model and already saw ourselves as predominantly a primary care provider—It was a good fit for the community." Others pointed to the regulatory flexibility that came with designation such as the flexibility in supervision and staffing. This was one of the key program-related reasons reported by CAHs located in frontier counties.

The majority of administrators reported that few hospital

operations and organisational relationships had changed solely because of participation in the Flex Programme. However, many of the administrators who originally felt the programme had not contributed to the changes their hospital had experienced since conversion later commented that those changes would not have been possible without the added resources and flexibility provided through programme participation (i.e., the changes would have occurred much later or perhaps not at all).

Strategic Related: Almost ten percent of the surveyed administrators identified strategic-related reasons for their hospital's conversion. Considering the overwhelming importance of finances and programme fit, this would seem to indicate the intent of some administrators to use the CAH conversion as an opportunity for proactive planning.

Some respondents reported that the conversion of their hospital was the result of an existing strategic plan—"We decided (to convert) during our strategic retreat," while others described less elaborate efforts that closely approximated the creation of a business plan. For one administrator the most important part of business plan development was the ongoing debate among the management team about the way the hospital should operate following conversion. He felt that it was critical to get expectations and assumptions out in the open and to discuss their merits relative to what could be expected of the CAH model. This provided a venue for identifying and avoiding market mistakes. For his hospital's conversion decision the final criterion was "if it doesn't make good business sense when you're not a CAH, it doesn't make good sense when you are one." He highly recommended use of this strategy by all CAH administrators. For these 10 percent, we begin to see the act of conversion as an enabling strategy rather than a reactionary strategy. Conversion is being used to position organisations for the next steps in a broader strategy to meet both existing and emerging market requirements, rather than as an end point for maintaining the status quo. In site visits, we heard many examples of actions to maintain the status quo, which is more familiar and comfortable than innovation, as well as appealing to the risk-averse.

Community Related: Only seven percent of the administrators in the survey identified community-related reasons for conversion. This is not surprising given the strong financial motivations for CAH conversion and the opportunity to list only two reasons as a rationale for conversion. Some spoke of reasons that were somewhat altruistic but also related to their survival, such as "keep health care in the community," while others focused more on the ethical and strategic aspects of community such as the "...community desires and deserves a strong array of services." Whether altruistic, strategic, or just sentimental, these and other comments clearly underscore the extent to which some of these hospitals are embedded in their local communities and are a part of the community's economic and social life.

Policy and Regulations: Surprisingly, few administrators identified existing or emerging rural health policy and regulations as one of their chief reasons for conversion to a CAH. It is possible that this finding reflects the historical trend that has been developing since the Balanced Budget Act (BBA) of 1997 was first passed (i.e., rescinding key financial provisions that adversely affected rural hospitals). It is also possible that much of the concern about the reimbursement and regulatory constraints spelled out in the BBA and retained in subsequent law was captured with statements about financial reasons for conversion.

INDUSTRY SNAPSHOT: HOSPITALS

This study describes how hospitals are paid, trends in hospital pricing, the pressures hospitals face, and delivery innovations, including hospital networks. This study considers a number of current controversies, including payor complaints that hospitals are exercising market power and hospital complaints about single- specialty hospitals. Representatives from hospitals and hospital organisations, as well as legal, economic, and academic experts, and government officials spoke at the Hearings. Hospital topic panels included Perspectives on Competition Policy and the Health Care Marketplace (February 27); A Tale of Two Cities (February 28, April 11); Hospital Round Table (March 26); Defining Product Markets for Hospitals (March 26); Defining Geographic Markets for Hospitals (March 26); Single Specialty Hospitals (March 27); Contracting Practices (March 27); Issues in Litigating Hospital Mergers (March 28); Hospitals—Horizontal Networks and Vertical Arrangements (April 9, 2003); Hospitals—Non-profit Status (April 10); Hospital Joint Ventures and Joint Operating Agreements (April 10); Hospitals—Post-Merger Conduct (April 11); Physician Hospital Organisations (May 8, 2003); Quality and Consumer Information: Hospitals (May 29); and Group Purchasing Organisations (September 26). Many industry representatives and experts also testified at the Commission's 2002 Health Care Workshop.

In cities and towns throughout the United States, hospitals are a key part of the health care delivery system. Hospitals are there when Americans give birth or die, are injured, or live with a chronic illness. Hospitals respond to the health care challenges in their communities, whether the problem is SARS or syphilis, anthrax or chicken pox, obesity or influenza. Hospitals provide care to the rich and poor, the well insured and the uninsured. Currently, payments to hospitals for inpatient care account for approximately 31 percent of total health care expenditures in the United States. The percentage of total expenditures devoted to inpatient care has declined over the past two decades, along with declines in hospital length-of-stay and the per capita rate of hospitalisation. During the period 1993-98, spending on hospital inpatient care increased by 3.4 percent per year. The past four years have seen annual increases that are double or triple that amount. Federal and state governments are responsible for almost 60 percent of payments to hospitals for inpatient care. For some services, the Centers for Medicare & Medicaid Services (CMS) is the sole payor. CMS's substantial share of hospital spending influences the rest of the financing and delivery markets for hospital services. Although CMS uses an administered pricing system for Medicare, hospitals engage in non-price competition to attract Medicare and Medicaid beneficiaries, and engage in price and non-price competition for private payors and patients. As detailed below, competition in the market for hospital inpatient services has enhanced quality and lowered prices. Private and public payors are encouraging these improvements by giving providers financial and nonfinancial incentives to increase quality and disseminate quality-related information to patients.

Description of Hospitals

Hospitals fall into one of three categories: (1) publicly owned hospitals, (2) nonprofit hospitals, and (3) for-profit hospitals. Although these classifications might appear distinct and immutable, they are not. Many nonprofit hospitals own for-profit institutions or have for-profit subsidiaries. For-profit systems manage nonprofit and publicly owned hospitals. Hospitals also may change their institutional status. One study demonstrated that over a thirteen year period, approximately one percent of hospitals changed their institutional status every year. Nonprofit hospitals currently make up about 61 percent of community hospitals and have roughly 71 percent of inpatient beds. For-profit hospitals comprise approximately 15 percent of community hospitals and 13 percent of inpatient beds. The remaining 24 percent of community hospitals are run by federal, state, and local governments, and account for 16 percent of inpatient beds. Hospitals are also frequently categorized as primary, secondary, tertiary, and quaternary, dependent on the level and complexity of care provided.

For example, a primary care hospital offers basic services such as an emergency department and limited intensive care facilities. A secondary care hospital generally offers primary care, general internal medicine, and limited surgical and diagnostic capabilities. A tertiary care hospital provides a full range of basic and sophisticated diagnostic and treatment services, including many specialized services.

A quaternary hospital typically provides sub-specialty services, such as advanced trauma care and organ transplantation. These distinctions, however, are not always clear in practice, as hospitals are not restricted to only offering the services associated with one category. Hospitals provide either general inpatient services or specialize in a particular kind of patient *(e.g.,* pediatric and women's hospitals) or condition *(e.g.,* cardiac, orthopedic, psychiatric and rehabilitation hospitals).

Regardless of how one categorizes private hospitals, they face similar market pressures and competitive constraints. Hospitals seek to provide cost-effective care and generate sufficient margins to continue to provide care to the community. Indeed, it is a misnomer to use the word "nonprofit;" as hospital administrators are fond of saying, "no margin, no mission."

How are Hospitals Paid: A Historical Perspective

Prior to 1983, Medicare and most other insurers paid hospitals on a cost-based reimbursement system. Under the cost-based reimbursement system, hospitals informed payors of the cost of the care that was provided, and those amounts were then paid. Although there were some constraints on how much a hospital could claim as its costs, the result was to reward volume and discourage efficiency. Payors picked up the cost of each service, each ordered test, and each day in the hospital. Additionally, comprehensive health insurance (both private and public) imposed minimal out-of-pocket costs on patients.

Thus, insured patients had little incentive to select lower cost procedures or more efficient providers. As a passive pay or of bills, the pay or had no control over expenditures. This payment system led to substantial increases in health care spending. Payors sought to curb these costs through various methods. Medicare implemented a prospective payment system in 1983, and has experimented with a range of strategies for creating incentives for hospitals to constrain their pricing. Private payors have done the same, in many instances piggybacking off strategies developed by CMS. Medicaid programmes have also adopted their own pricing strategies. The rise of managed care and other delivery-side innovations have also had a significant impact on hospital pricing.

A. Public Payors

The most significant public payor is CMS, which administers the Medicare and Medicaid programmes. In 1983, Congress directed CMS largely to abandon cost-based reimbursement for acute inpatient care delivered to Medicare beneficiaries, and adopt the inpatient prospective payment system (IPPS). The IPPS was intended to moderate the rising federal expenditures, create a more "competitive, market-like environment, and ... curb inefficiencies in hospital operations engendered by reimbursement of incurred cost." Under the IPPS, the amount a hospital receives for treating a patient is based on the diagnosis-related group (DRG) for the episode of hospitalisation. The DRG assigned to a particular episode of hospitalisation is based on the diagnosis at discharge that justified the hospitalisation. Each DRG has a payment weight assigned to it, based on the average cost of treating patients in that DRG. The average DRG cost reflects both the very ill patients that require more intensive care and the "healthy" ill who do not cost as much to treat. Hospitals receive this predetermined amount regardless of the actual cost of care.

Certain hospitals receive an adjusted payment in excess of the standard DRG amount. Teaching hospitals and hospitals treating a disproportionate share of low-income patients receive higher payments. All DRGs include a wage index, tied to the geographic location of the hospital. Moreover, if the treatment of a particular patient is exceptionally costly, an "outlier" adjustment is added. Prior to August 1, 2000, CMS paid hospitals for outpatient care on a cost-based system. Since that date, hospitals, pursuant to the Balanced Budget Act of 1997, are paid for outpatient care under the outpatient prospective payment system (OPPS). Under OPPS, hospitals receive a predetermined amount for all outpatient services or procedures, based on which one of the approximately 750 ambulatory payment classifications (APCs) the episode of care falls into. The OPPS encompasses all evaluation and management services and procedures provided by hospitals on an outpatient basis. For example, the APC for a particular outpatient surgical procedure includes payment for all operating and recovery room services, anesthesia, and surgical supplies. Each APC is assigned a general weight based on the median cost of providing the service.

Effective October 1, 2000, Medicare adopted a prospective payment system for home health care services. Moreover, as of 2007, Medicare is scheduled to begin employing a competitive bidding system to determine which providers will offer durable medical equipment to Medicare beneficiaries. The IPPS system was designed to control rising inpatient hospital costs and shift more care to the outpatient setting. The OPPS was designed to control rising outpatient costs. Both systems constrained costs more effectively than the cost-based systems they replaced. Because the government establishes prices in the IPPS and OPPS, neither system adequately reflects the prices that would prevail in a competitive market. Each state also has a Medicaid programme, which pays for care provided to the poor and disabled. Within broad guidelines established by Federal law, each state sets its own payment rate for Medicaid services and administers its own programme. Medicaid programmes either pay health care providers directly on a fee-for-service basis, or use prepayment arrangements such as health maintenance organisations (HMOs). Many states have aggressively adopted prepayment arrangements for the Medicaid population.

B. Private Payors

In some instances, private payors copied the reimbursement strategies of the Medicare programme, or used Medicare DRGs as a reference price for negotiation. Thus, some payors negotiate either a specified discount or a specified payment relative to the amount CMS would pay for a specified treatment episode. More often, private payors and hospitals negotiate discounts from charges *(e.g.,* they pay 85 percent of billed charges) or a per diem rate. Some contracts provide for a fixed payment for inpatient services on a per-case basis. Outpatient payment provisions are typically structured on a percentage-of-billed charges or fee-schedule basis.

Rising Hospital Prices

Expenditures on hospital services have grown over the past two decades, but the rate of spending growth has varied. As noted previously, IPPS slowed the rate of hospital expenditure growth. The rise of managed care slowed the rate of expenditure growth further; from 1993 through 1998, hospital expenditures increased at an average annual rate of 3.7 percent and in some areas of the country, the per diem price of a hospital stay actually decreased. In the past five years, rising hospital prices have driven spending on hospitals higher, even though hospital utilisation is declining.

Analysts attribute rising hospital prices to a variety of factors including "hospitals' increasing ability to negotiate higher prices from private payers." Two recent studies project spending on inpatient hospital services will continue to increase in the coming decade. CMS estimated that expenditures on inpatient care will grow at an average rate of 6.4 percent per year until 2005, and then grow at a slower rate of 5.6 percent through 2013. Thus, spending on hospital care is estimated to total $934 billion in 2013, or a 55 percent real increase per capita. These estimates are premised on the expectation that rising health care costs and a slowing economy will make employers and consumers more willing to accept restrictions on coverage. Similarly, another paper projected expenditures on hospital services will increase by 75 percent per capita. Thus, experts predict spending on inpatient care will increase much faster than inflation in the coming decade.

Pressures on Hospitals

Panelists listed a number of pressures facing hospitals. These pressures included increasing costs from the public's demand for the latest technology, the aging of the population, shortages of nursing staff and other hospital personnel (which have forced hospitals to increase salaries), increased regulatory requirements, payor demands for information, patient safety initiatives, meeting homeland security requirements, the rising cost of liability premiums and prescription drugs, and the obligation of providing care to the uninsured. Hospital representatives also emphasized the impact of managed care and the cuts imposed by the Balanced Budget Act of 1997 on reimbursement. Panelists asserted that these pressures explained and justified recent hospital price increases.

Reorganisation of the Hospital System

Over the past 20 years, hospitals have been consolidating into multi-hospital systems. In 2001, almost 54 percent of hospitals operated as part of a system, with an additional 12.7 percent working in looser health networks. In 1979, only about 31 percent of hospitals were part of a system. Consolidation presents an opportunity for hospitals to compete more efficiently. Consolidated hospitals can employ mechanisms to improve the quality of care and limit duplication of services or administrative expenses. Consolidated hospitals may also be able to improve quality if they centralize performance of complex procedures for which greater volume leads to higher quality. Consolidated hospitals could also use their combined resources to track established clinical quality measures and develop new ones. Initially, national systems acquired hospitals throughout the United States, but recent acquisitions have been more localized. For example, according to one panelist, St. Louis has 31 hospitals. Four of those hospitals are independent;

the remaining hospitals have joined one of four local systems. Similarly, one academic described the consolidation in San Francisco: by 1999 "almost all hospitals ... became part of one of four not-for-profit hospital systems." Another panelist described the Boston metropolitan area consolidation as being one where "through mergers and acquisitions ... the PCHI [Partners Community HealthCare Inc.] network now numbers 15 hospitals and more than 5,000 physicians." One study noted dramatic consolidation in numerous communities, including Cleveland, "where two local hospital systems now control nearly 70 percent of the area's inpatient capacity," and Indianapolis and Phoenix, where "hospitals have carved out strongholds in key urban and suburban areas, at times creating virtual monopolies in geographic submarkets." Hospitals may consolidate within a single market or across markets, and consolidation can occur over a broad spectrum of possibilities. At one end of the spectrum, consolidating hospitals have a shared license and common ownership, report unified financial records, and eliminate duplicative facilities. At the other end of the spectrum, a common governing body owns the consolidating hospitals, but the hospitals maintain separate hospital facilities, retain their individual business licenses, and keep separate financial records. Hospital systems have varying degrees of centralized control. One panelist noted that some systems have a parent organisation that sets policy and makes key decisions. At the other extreme, the same panelist noted that some systems offer little more than centralized administrative oversight and capital financing. Another panelist noted that "the various hospital mergers that were particularly frequent in the mid-1990s tended not to follow through when it came to clinical integration .."

Panelists identified several reasons for hospital consolidation, including the reduction of excess capacity, the rise of managed care, increased ability to assume capitated financial risk, expansion of the hospital's delivery network, and service consolidation and coordination.Analysts have also suggested other factors that might be driving consolidation, including the desire to obtain economies of scale in purchasing or production, access to capital markets, and "specialisation in labor or management techniques."

Some panelists assert hospital consolidation has promoted efficiency, led to savings, and instilled life back into failing hospitals. Other panelists believe the primary result of consolidation has been the creation of hospital market power against payors. One study examining consolidation through mergers found that hospitals that merged tended to be in less-concentrated markets and in areas with higher HMO penetration. Merging hospitals were also more likely to have been a member of a system, were larger, had higher occupancy rates and case-mix indexes, and higher pre-merger expenses and revenues.

One recent review examined the operational consequences of hospital consolidation. It found that when hospitals that consolidated were geographically distant, they generally had similar staffing ratios, similar occupancy rates, and substantial service duplication. For these distant hospitals, typically both were financially viable. Duplicative acute care services were generally not eliminated, unless one of the hospitals was more specialized, was economically weaker or had different staffing levels, or there existed a substantial degree of competition between the merging hospitals. One recent study indicated that when systems acquired hospitals, efficiencies did not materialize, because of the failure to combine operations.

Most studies of the relationship between competition and hospital prices generally find increased hospital concentration is associated with increased prices. One study found that merged hospitals experience larger price and cost increases than those that have not merged, except in less concentrated areas where these patterns were reversed. Another study using similar data and methods found that merger cost and price savings were lower than the first study when merging hospitals were compared against rival institutions. One set of commentators has observed that most empirical studies on concentration and consolidation do not differentiate among transactions that occur within markets and those that occur across markets, even though these transactions "might reflect very different hospital strategies and consequently, could have different effects on efficiency." According to several panelists, hospital systems try to make sure they have at least one "must have" hospital in each geographic market in which they compete. A "must have" hospital or hospital system is one that health care plans believe they must offer to their beneficiaries to attract employers to their plan. According to some panelists, this status allows the hospital or hospital system to demand price increases.

Consolidation has resulted in complaints by payors about the exercise of market power by hospitals. Some panelists and commentators believe an important motivation for the creation of multi-hospital systems has been to gain market power to secure higher reimbursement from payors. One panelist stated the various hospital mergers occurring in the mid-1990s "tended not to follow through when it came to clinical integration and ultimately providers have regained the leverage with health plans that they had lost." Another study examined the relationship between market power and pricing in nonprofit, multi-hospital systems. The investigation led to two primary findings: (1) nonprofit hospitals that were members of national or regional systems appear to have priced their services "more aggressively in the presence of market power" than the hospitals did when operating independently or as members of local systems; and (2) nonprofit systems showed a tendency to exercise market power in the form of higher prices. The rise of hospital systems has affected market concentration in certain markets. One study found that if hospital system members within metropolitan statistical areas (MSA) are treated as one entity, nineteen MSAs became concentrated between 1995 and 2000. Seven of the 19 MSAs showed an increase in HHI of at least 1,700. As discussed in this study, the Agencies will continue to evaluate hospital consolidation to determine whether consolidation (or potential consolidation) in any given market is anticompetitive.

The Impact of Government Purchasing

CMS has tremendous bargaining power in the market for medical services, and providers are extremely responsive to the signals sent by CMS. Prior to the adoption of the IPPS, average hospital length-of-stay had been stable for 7 years. Once IPPS went into effect, length of stay began an immediate decline, the number of inpatient cataract surgeries dropped precipitously (from 630,000 to 211,000 in one year), and the number of hospital outpatient cataract surgeries immediately increased by 128 percent. Similarly, the adoption of prospective payment for home health care had an immediate impact on the number of beneficiaries that received services and the average number of visits.

Medicare's administered pricing system can also (albeit generally inadvertently) make some services extraordinarily lucrative, and others unprofitable. The result of the pricing distortions is that some services are more or less available than they would be based on the demand for the services—which in turn triggers adaptive responses by providers.

One panelist noted these difficulties are compounded by the fact that the balance of the population relies for its health care services on an infrastructure built in response to the excesses and inadequacies of Medicare's administered pricing system.

Consider cardiac care. Commentators and panelists suggested that CMS never made a deliberate decision to provide for greater profits for such services relative to the amounts paid for other inpatient services but the IPPS does so. General hospitals use these profits to subsidize the provision of less profitable (or unprofitable) services, but the pricing distortion creates a direct economic incentive for SSHs to enter the market. In response, general hospitals complain to legislators and try to find ways to limit the expansion of competition. Absent the distortions created by the excess profits for cardiac services in Medicare's administered pricing system, the incentive for SSH entry would be less. These difficulties are magnified when the government is the sole or primary purchaser of a good or service. Paying too much wastes resources, while paying too little reduces both output and capacity, lowers the quality of the services that are provided, and diminishes the incentives for innovation. Some commentators have suggested that these adverse consequences have materialized in the market for vaccines.

Although CMS can set prices, there are limitations to CMS's ability to create incentives that encourage price and non-price competition among providers. CMS does not have the freedom to respond as a private purchaser would to changes in the marketplace. For example, CMS has only limited authority to contract selectively with providers or to use competitive bidding to meet its needs. With limited exceptions, CMS cannot force providers to compete for CMS's business or encourage suppliers to reduce their costs and enhance their quality by rewarding them with substantially increased volume or substantially higher payments if they do. Even straightforward purchasing initiatives, such as competitive bidding for durable medical equipment (DME), have generated considerable resistance. A pilot project resulted in Medicare savings between 17 and 22 percent with no significant adverse effects on beneficiaries. Opponents of competitive bidding have argued, however, that the bidding process increased bureaucracy, decreased consumer choice, threatened the existence of small manufacturers, and lowered quality. At least one industry representative has called for the repeal of the provisions mandating competitive bidding.

With limited exceptions, CMS's payment systems do not reward higher quality care, or punish lower quality care. Indeed, as the Medicare Payment Advisory Commission (MedPAC) noted, the Medicare payment system is "largely neutral or negative towards quality. All providers meeting basic requirements are paid the same regardless of the quality of service provided. At times providers are paid even more when quality is worse, such as when the complications occur as the result of error." Former CMS administrator Scully was more pointed: Medicare pays every hospital in a region "the exact same amount for hip replacement and the same amount for a heart bypass, if you're the best hospital or the worst hospital."

To be sure, these problems are not unique to Medicare. The Institute of Medicine noted that "current [compensation] methods provide little financial reward for improvements in the quality of health care delivery, and may even inadvertently pose barriers to innovation." The Agencies encourage the use of payment strategies that create an incentive for providers to deliver higher quality care to consumers. Medicare also includes a managed care option, the Medicare Advantage (MA) programme. MA programmes provide Medicare beneficiaries with a range of managed care options, including HMOs and preferred provider organisations. MA allows Medicare beneficiaries to join privately operated managed care plans.

The plans are paid an administratively determined rate by Medicare and plans also may charge an additional premium and offer additional benefits. Medicare beneficiaries who joined MA plans often received greater benefits *(e.g.,* prescription drug coverage) in exchange for accepting limits on their choice of providers. In 2002, MA plans (then the Medicare+Choice (M+C) plan) provided health care to 5 million Medicare beneficiaries, down from 6.35 million enrollees in December 1999. One panelist testified that although the Medicare programme has attempted to introduce competitive pricing as a way to set payment rates to M+C plans, to date none of those plans have been successful. As a result, Medicare continues to establish the payment rates administratively. According to this speaker, to the extent plans compete, it typically has been on the benefits they provide.

Entry of Speciality Hospitals and Ambulatory Surgery Centres

Specialty hospitals provide care for a specific specialty *(e.g.,* cardiac, orthopedic, or psychiatric) or type of patient *(e.g.,* children or women). Specialty hospitals tailor their care and facilities to fit the chosen type of condition, patient, or procedure on which they focus. Specialty hospitals are not new to the hospital industry. Pediatric and psychiatric hospitals have existed for decades. More recently, numerous cardiac and orthopedic surgery hospitals have opened or are under construction. These single-specialty hospitals (SSHs) differ from their predecessors in that many of the physicians who refer patients have an ownership interest in the facility. SSHs may compete with both inpatient and outpatient general hospital surgery departments as well as with ambulatory surgery centers.

There are relatively few SSHs. In October 2003, the General Accounting Office identified 100 existing SSHs with an additional 26 under development. SSHs are located in 28 states, but two-thirds are located in only seven states. The GAO concluded that "the location of specialty hospitals is strongly correlated to whether states allow hospitals to add beds or build new facilities without first obtaining state approval for such health care capacity increases."Ninety-six percent of the opened SSHs and all 26 SSHs under development are located in such states. The recently imposed moratorium on Medicare payments to SSHs, and the results of two Congressionally mandated studies on the industry are likely to affect the future development of these hospitals. Under the moratorium, physicians may not refer Medicare patients to a specialty hospital in which they have an ownership interest, and Medicare may not pay specialty hospitals for any services rendered as a result of a prohibited referral.

Panelists identified a number of market developments that encouraged the emergence of SSHs, including: less tightly managed care; the willingness of providers to invest in a SSH;physicians' desire to "provide better, more timely patient care"; physicians looking for ways to supplement declining professional fees; and the growth of entrepreneurial firms, such as MedCath and National Surgical Hospitals. Panelists also stated that some providers desire greater control over management decisions that affect their incomes and productivity. Several panelists suggested efficiency was an important consideration for many providers: specialty hospitals allow "surgeons to start on time, do more cases in a given amount of time, and get back to their office on time." One panelist asserted that physicians view SSHs as a "a blank slate" and an "opportunity to make improvements in the care delivery process" by "redesign[ing] the care delivery process in a way to be more effective and efficient."

Several panelists contended that SSHs achieve better outcomes through increased volume, better disease management, and better clinical standards. They attribute these positive outcomes to their focus on a single specialty. For example, MedCath stated that its focus has allowed it to increase access to cardiac monitored beds, "improve access to emergency services," "improve clinical outcomes" and lower the cost of care by having shorter hospital stays, discharging a higher percentage of patients directly home, and using the nursing labor pool efficiently.

A panelist representing MedCath presented a study showing that 90 percent of its patients were discharged directly to home, compared to "72 percent for the peer community hospitals and 70 percent for the teaching facilities." According to this panelist, for each early discharge, MedCath hospitals saved "Medicare over $1,000 per discharge." Other panelists stated that physician-investors send healthier, lower-risk patients to the SSH and sicker patients to the general hospital. Several panelists argued that this allows SSHs "to produce service less expensively, while often being paid the same or more than community hospitals." An April, 2003 GAO report found that patients at specialty hospitals tended to be less sick than patients with the same diagnoses at general hospitals.

Similarly, several panelists noted that some SSHs do not provide emergency departments and thus avoid the higher costs of trauma treatment and indigent care. Those panelists believe this gives SSHs an unfair competitive advantage over 24-hour hospitals with emergency departments. The October 2003 GAO study analysed whether

SSHs provided care to Medicare and Medicaid patients and had emergency departments. As Table 1 shows, the study found that there were modest differences between the percentage of Medicare and Medicaid patients who received treatment at general hospitals and SSHs.

TABLE 1

	General Hospitals	*Specialty Hospitals*
Orthopedic Medicaid Admissions	10%	8%
Cardiac Care Medicaid Admissions	6%	3%
Medicaid Admissions for Women's Health	37%	28%

One panelist observed that general hospitals are reluctant to have their performance compared to specialty providers who do not handle the same case mix or have the same cost structures. Some panelists argued that the SSHs and ambulatory surgery centers are inherently risky for patients with multiple conditions. They argued that chronic disease management, rather than fragmented specialty services, will serve those patients better. Several panelists were concerned that SSHs would siphon off the most profitable procedures and patients, leaving general hospitals with less money to cross subsidize other socially valuable, but less profitable, care. As one panelist stated, "it is the profitable services they are taking away that jeopardizes a hospital's capability of providing unprofitable services." Panelists expressed concern that "the community [will] lose[] access to specific services or ultimately to all hospital services as the general hospital deteriorates or closes." Several panelists also suggested that physicians that have an ownership interest in a SSH have an incentive to over-refer patients to that facility to maximise their income.

The GAO summarized these competing perspectives on SSHs:

> Advocates of these hospitals contend that the focused mission and dedicated resources of specialty hospitals both improve quality and reduce costs. Critics contend that specialty hospitals siphon off the most profitable procedures and patient cases, thus eroding the financial health of neighboring general hospitals and impairing their ability to provide emergency care and other essential community services.

Market Reaction to SSH Entry. *According to several panelists, some general hospitals facing competition from SSHs have removed the admitting privileges of physicians involved with a specialty hospital. Several panelists stated that such strategies are used to protect the viability of the general hospital and to avoid the conflict of interest that arises from a physician ownership interest in a facility to which they are referring patients. These panelists do not believe that removing the hospital privileges of physician-investors harms competition, and suggest that a hospital is not required "to sacrifice the interests of [its] charitable institution in favour of the physician's self-interest."*

Panelists also described a number of other responses by general hospitals to the emergence of SSHs. One panelist stated that some general hospitals have established their own specialized single-specialty wing or partnered with physicians on their medical staff to open a SSH. Panelists also stated that some general hospitals have reacted to the competition by removing physicians from the on-call rotation; making scheduling surgeries more difficult; limiting physician access to operating rooms; limiting physicians' "extra assignments" under which the physician can earn professional fees; and using certificate of need laws to encumber specialty hospital entry. Panelists also stated that general hospitals have entered into managed care contracts with health plans that either preclude SSH entry entirely, or result in the "deselection" of physicians who invest in the SSH from the insurance companies' list of preferred providers. Representatives of SSHs noted that it is difficult to compete against this behaviour by providing lower prices because they cannot provide the full panoply of services a health plan requires. One panelist summarized the SSH position as follows: general hospitals have engaged in "stiff and coordinated resistence ... driven not by quality, cost efficiency, or the desire to preserve the delivery of charity care to the community, but rather by the fear of having to compete, of having to look within their respective institutions to improve efficiencies and to enhance the timely delivery of patient care."

Ambulatory Surgery Centers. *Ambulatory surgery centers (ASCs) perform surgical procedures on patients who do not require an overnight stay in the hospital. Approximately half of the ASCs are single-specialty. Single-specialty ASCs generally specialize in either gastroenterology, orthopedics, or ophthalmology. Most ASCs are small (two to four operating rooms). ASCs' ownership structures vary: some are completely physician owned; some are owned by joint ventures between physicians and private or publicly traded companies; some are owned by physician / hospital joint ventures; and some are owned by hospitals and hospital networks. Innovations in technology have made it possible to offer a broad range of services in ASCs.*

ASCs require less capital than SSHs, and are generally less complex to develop because they do not require the facilities needed to offer care twenty-four hours a day, seven days a week. ASCs generally do not have emergency departments, and certificate of need regulations often are not as rigorous for ASCs, if they apply at all. ASCs were originally intended to compete with hospital inpatient units, but they now compete more against hospital outpatient surgery units. The number of ASCs has doubled in the past decade, and currently total 3,371. Panelists indicated ASC development was influenced by many of the same factors spurring the growth of specialty hospitals. One panelist noted that ASCs were "a common-sense, intelligent response to a mature health care delivery system and industry gripped by inefficiencies and to health care spending being out of control." Other reasons for ASC growth listed by panelists included improved technology, physician demand for efficient surgical facilities, control and specialized staff, as well as "patient demand for a non-institutional, friendly, convenient setting for their surgical care, and payor demand for cost efficiencies as evidenced by the ambulatory surgery center industry." One study also noted that ASCs offer patients more "convenient locations, shorter wait times, and lower coinsurance than a hospital department."

Medicare reimbursement has had a profound impact on the number of ASCs and the amount of surgery performed in them. Congress first approved coverage of ASCs by Medicare in 1980, as part of an effort to control health care spending by providing low-risk surgeries in a less-expensive ambulatory setting. Between 1982 and 1988, Medicare paid 100 percent of the reasonable charges for approved ambulatory procedures, and waived the deductible and copayment that would apply if the procedure were provided in an inpatient setting. From 1988 to 2003, the fee schedule has been based on an inflation-adjusted 1986 cost survey for ambulatory surgery. The ASC payment schedule has not been adjusted for advances in technology and productivity over the last 16 years; some procedures that were once labor-and-resource intensive are now much less costly for ASCs to perform. The MMA freezes Medicare payment rates for ASCs from 2005 through 2009 and directs the

Department of Health and Human Services to implement a new payment system by 2008.

Although ASCs and hospital outpatient departments perform some of the same procedures, payment varies depending on where the services are provided. Higher reimbursement for services performed in a hospital outpatient department may make sense when a patient has multiple complicating factors making the surgery more complex. One panelist also asserted that hospitals should receive higher payments for outpatient services because they have higher overhead costs. Yet, as Table 2 demonstrates, payment may be higher, lower, or the same at ASCs and hospital outpatient departments. These differences create predictable incentives for providers.

TABLE 2

Medicare Reimbursement Rates for Procedures Performed by Hospital Outpatient Department and ASCs

Description	*Hospital Outpatient Rate*	*ASC Rate Difference*	*Percent*
Cataract removal/lens insertion	$1,160	$973	-19%
After cataract laser surgery	246	446	81
Colonoscopy, diagnostic	413	446	8
Upper gastrointestinal endoscopy, biopsy	387	446	15
Colonoscopy with removal of lesion by snare	413	446	8
Epidural injection, lumbar or sacral	250	333	33
Colonoscopy with biopsy	413	446	8
Colonoscopy with removal of lesion by forceps	413	446	8
Upper gastrointestinal endoscopy, diagnostic	387	333	-14
Cystoscopy	329	333	1

As former CMS administrator Tom Scully noted, when the ASC rate is high "all of a sudden you start seeing ASCs pop up all over the place to do colonoscopies or to do outpatient surgery .... If the hospitals get paid a little more, they're going to have more outpatient centers."

Many of the concerns expressed by panelists about SSHs were also expressed about ASCs. Panelists asserted that ASCs are eroding the outpatient market share of hospitals that hospitals depend upon, that ASCs do not care for Medicaid beneficiaries, they "skim and cherry-pick on the front end regarding [] the finances of the patient," and that ASCs only enter areas where business is profitable. One ASC representative suggested that reimbursement should be modified based on the acuity of the patient, but denied that ASCs refuse to care for Medicaid patients.

Market Reaction to ASC Entry. *Panelists indicated that many of the actions taken to curb entry of specialty hospitals are also being employed against ASCs. One panelist suggested that entry and competition for ASCs have been made difficult by hospitals engaging in legislative efforts to encumber ASCs with unnecessary regulation and mandatory services. Another panelist described how some hospitals have negotiated discounted prices for inpatient services in exchange for exclusive contracts for outpatient surgery. One panelist noted that some general hospitals have revoked privileges of physician-investors in ASCs, and used state certificate of need (CON) laws to inhibit ASC entry.*

Competitive Evaluation of Entry. *In general, the Agencies favour the elimination of anticompetitive barriers to entry, on the grounds that robustly competitive markets in which entry and exit is determined by market forces maximises consumer welfare. Entry by SSHs and ASCs has had a number of beneficial consequences for consumers who receive care from these providers. It cannot be overlooked, however, that Medicare's administered pricing system has substantially driven the emergence of SSHs and ASCs.*

Generally speaking, antitrust law does not limit individual hospitals from unilaterally responding to competition either by terminating physician admitting privileges or by approaching state governments in connection with CON proceedings. If there is specific evidence of anticompetitive conduct by individual hospitals or of hospitals colluding together against efforts to open a SSH or ASC, then the Agencies will aggressively pursue those activities.

Hospital/Payor Contracting in the Private Market

Contracting between hospitals and private payors has been controversial and contentious. Several panelists asserted that hospital systems routinely "terminate then negotiate" for large increases in reimbursement, and use the media to scare the public. Panelists also stated that hospital systems insist that all hospitals in the system be included in a payor network ("all or nothing contracts"), irrespective of whether the payor actually wants to include the entirety of the hospital system. Panelists representing hospitals responded that they are protecting their institutions' interests and that their services had been artificially and unsustainably underpriced in the past. These dynamics have played out in several markets in the past few years. Although commentators have noted that particular hospitals and systems seem to have the upper hand in some markets, whether hospitals or health plans have bargaining advantages varies substantially within and among different markets.

Generally speaking, payors seek to contract with hospitals that contribute to the marketability of their insurance products. Factors that affect marketability include the price of coverage, the number of hospitals at which care can be provided, the perceived quality, desirability, and accessibility of those institutions, and the alternative insurance products that are available in the market. Payors seek to balance the price of the hospital services they must purchase to offer insurance coverage against the desirability of the resulting network to the purchasers of their insurance products. If patients view several hospitals as adequate substitutes for one another, it will be easier for the payor to threaten credibly to exclude one or more of these hospitals. Conversely, if enrollees will drop an insurance plan if their preferred hospital is no longer in the network, the hospital will find it easier to insist on higher reimbursement. Multi-hospital systems frequently seek to ensure that all system hospitals are included in a payor network. Consumer pressure for open networks has made it more difficult for payors to exclude an entire hospital system outright, which affects the bargaining dynamics.

In a few markets, payors have sought to "tier" hospitals. Tiering results in different consumer copayments *(i.e.,* high or low cost sharing) depending on the hospital at which care is provided. Hospital tiers may be established using a wide variety of criteria. Tiering generally does not apply to emergency admissions, and may depend upon where routine and specialty services are offered. For payors, tiering offers a potential response to multi-hospital system pressure for inclusion of all system hospitals within a payor network.

Tiering allows the payor to maintain a broad network, and include a "must-have" hospital, but simultaneously creates an incentive for consumers to use lower-cost providers. Panelists offered a range of views on the prospects of tiering. Blue Shield of California provides one example of tiered hospital benefits. Blue Shield tiers within geographic areas and seeks to promote choice among community hospitals and teaching hospitals.

Hospitals are sorted by region and teaching status and coverage benefits are designed to operate within these groupings. Blue Shield also uses some quality performance measures in its tiering criteria. Hospitals are assigned to a "choice" tier unless their prices exceed the average for their region and teaching status, in which case they are assigned to an "affiliate" tier. Blue Shield introduced this product in April 2002. Approximately, one million of its 2.3 million members have a tiered network benefit package. Blue Shield tiers inpatient and outpatient services, ambulatory surgery centers, and radiation and chemotherapy services.

Similarly, Tufts Health Plan also attempted to use tiering in Boston, Massachusetts.Teaching hospitals provide the majority of hospital services within Boston and are typically more expensive than community hospitals. Tufts tried to use tiering to steer its members to community hospitals. After a very public battle, Tufts backed away from its plans and made tiering voluntary for its members.

Some hospitals resist tiering, and if they have sufficient bargaining power, they can credibly threaten to withdraw from a pay or network if they are placed in an unfavourable tier. Hospital systems can similarly threaten to pull all of their hospitals from a network if any system hospital is placed in an unfavourable tier. In some markets, hospital systems have taken preemptive steps to negotiate contract language with plans that prohibit tiering. Panelists and analysts noted a number of reasons (beyond straight financial issues) why hospitals may resist tiering. Low-cost facilities fear being labeled as low quality and high-cost facilities fear being deemed inefficient. If tiering is price-driven, it may be difficult for facilities to maintain expensive areas of care like burn units, trauma services, and emergency "standby" capabilities.Hospital representatives also expressed concern that individual hospitals are not fungible substitutes, and tiering might result in bad consumer choices. Hospital representatives have also expressed concern that tiering might force poor consumers to patronize only low-quality, low-cost hospitals. One critic of hospital tiering believes that tiering will put indigent care, teaching facilities, and innovative research at risk, and believes "there is no justification for putting patients in the middle of ... health care financing"—particularly when the available information about quality is less than perfect.

Because tiering is a relatively new development, there are no systematic studies available on the prevalence or consequences of this strategy. Additional research would be useful in determining whether consumers in tiered plans actually use lower priced hospitals, and whether they would have used those hospitals without the tiering.

Hospital Pricing: Distinguishing Among Bulk Pruchasing, Price Discrimination, Costing Shifting, and Corss Subsidies

Understanding hospital pricing requires an understanding of four terms: bulk purchasing, price discrimination, cost shifting, and cross subsidies. The terms have distinct meanings, although there is some overlap between cost shifting and cross subsidies. Bulk purchasing usually occurs when large organisations *(e.g.,* insurance companies) receive purchasing discounts because of the volume of their purchases. This type of purchasing can help reduce the cost of health care because the bulk purchasing capability can be used to obtain a large discount. For example, insurance companies often secure better hospital care rates for their beneficiaries than uninsured individual may obtain. There is nothing unusual about this behaviour and it has a long history in commercial practice, in the courts, and in economic analysis. The conventional definition of price discrimination is different ratios of price (P) to marginal cost (MC) for the same service across different buyers. That is P/MC for consumer "j" is not equal to P/MC for consumer "k". For example, senior citizens may pay less to watch the same movie at the same time as other adults. Like bulk purchasing, price discrimination has a long history in commercial practice, in the courts, and in economic analysis.

Cost shifting refers to raising the price charged to one group of consumers as a result of lowering the price to other consumers. An example would be a hospital raising the price to privately insured patients because the government lowered the price it paid for Medicare patients. The hospital raises the privately insured prices closer to the profit maximising level. There are three essential elements to cost shifting: (1) the company or hospital must have market power that it has not exploited; (2) in response to a pay or lowering its price, the company raises its prices to other payers; and (3) the ability to cost-shift is limited by the profit maximising price. Some economists will concede that cost-shifting may exist as a matter of theory for non-profit maximising firms, but question whether it actually occurs.

Cross subsidizing is the practice of charging supracompetitive prices to some payors or for some services and using the surpluses to subsidize other payors or other clinical services. Cross subsidisation is similar to cost shifting in that it can occur if a non-profit-maximising firm has market power. Cross-subsidies can occur if there are barriers to entry in a market and a nonprofit-maximising firm receives greater profits on some services *(e.g.,* from Medicare for cardiac services) that it uses to underwrite the provision of other services. In a competitive market, such cross-subsidies are competed away. Hospital panelists see cross subsidies not as a theory, but as a fact of life:

[If we] take away those profitable services and leave

the hospital, the community hospital, with just the unprofitable services, one of two things is going to happen. Either services will be diminished to the community in a way that is not transparent, in a way that they cannot see that happening, or costs will be shifted back to other payors, and business and labor and consumers end up absorbing them, once again, not in a transparent way where they can see what's happening.

As noted previously, Congress has created direct subsidies for certain hospitals. CMS pays more (approximately $5.9 billion extra in 1999) to teaching hospitals and it pays more (approximately $5 billion per year) to safety net hospitals that provide a disproportionate share of care to the poor. More recently, the MMA includes a provision for $250 million in extra payments to hospitals in states that border Mexico, to pay for the costs of providing emergency care to undocumented aliens.

Reliance on cross-subsidies, instead of direct subsidies, to ensure access to care makes the availability of such care contingent on the location in which care is provided, the wealth and insurance status of those receiving care at any given hospital, and the un-competitiveness of the market for hospital services. Several panelists noted that in some communities, hospitals make substantial profits on one group and use those funds to provide charity care to the balance of the community. In other locations, this approach is not viable—particularly if those paying the bills identify alternative locations to provide care that choose not to engage in cross subsidisation. Cross subsidies distort relative prices, resulting in inefficient decisions by payors and patients. Cross subsidies also complicate attempts to provide consumers with better price information. Finally, it is generally more efficient to subsidize directly, rather than pay higher prices elsewhere and cross subsidize.

Consumer Price Sensitivity and Information

Tiering represents an attempt to force consumers to bear some of the increased price associated with receiving care at a more expensive hospital. Medical savings accounts are intended to accomplish the same goal. That is, both strategies attempt to raise consumer sensitivity to the costs associated with the health care decisions. For these strategies to work effectively, however, consumers will need access to good information about the price and quality of the services they must choose between. A consumer facing a 25 percent co-payment at one hospital and a 15 percent co-payment at another can not accurately assess the financial consequences of choosing one hospital over the other absent good information about the price of the services that will be rendered at both hospitals. Most insured consumers are "rationally ignorant" of the price of the medical services they receive, because insurance largely insulates them from the financial implications of their medical treatment.

Consumers who pay the same co-payment regardless of the price of the treatment they receive have no reason to inquire into the price of the treatment, or to factor that price into their decision. Consumers who have co-payments that vary depending on where they receive care will still focus on the amount of the co-payment, and not on the total price of the services they receive. Even if consumers are interested in knowing the total price of the care they receive, they would find it extremely difficult to obtain that information, and are likely to find it to be complicated and obscure. Proposals to increase consumer price sensitivity must confront this reality, and develop strategies to increase the transparency of hospital pricing. To be sure, these difficulties do not apply to payors, who deal with multiple providers in multiple geographic and product markets, and use pricing information to make contracting decisions.

Cross Subsidies and Competition

As noted previously, cross subsidies require either the exercise of market power by a non-profit-maximising firm, or a non-profit-maximising firm that receives supra-competitive profits on some services in a market with barriers to entry. As competition becomes more effective in hospital markets, these cross subsidies will tend to be competed away.

Competition can help make health care more affordable, but it cannot transfer resources to those who do not have them. SSHs and ASCs may well enhance quality of care, lower prices, and improve access. From the perspective of those receiving care at the SSH or ASC, that is a desirable outcome. From the perspective of the general hospital that relied on specialty care to cross subsidize unprofitable patients and services, and from the perspective of such patients and perhaps others that the hospital serves, the same outcome is undesirable.

Competition has a number of effects on hospitals, including the potential to improve quality and lower costs. Competition will also undermine the ability of hospitals to engage in cross-subsidisation, however. To address this issue, Congress and state legislatures should consider whether direct subsidies for desired conduct are advisable.

HOSPITAL ADMISSIONS

The most important right of a member of a hospital medical staff is the right to admit patients to the hospital. The admission of a patient of a patient to a hospital requires decisions by both the admitting physician and the hospital administrator (in the latter case the decisions being usually delegated to an admitting clerk). The interaction of these two decision makers may have serious consequences that must be considered in the medical quality control programme. The most common conflict arises when the admitting clerk declines to admit a patient that the physician has ordered to be admitted. The usual reason is that the patient is unable to pay for the hospitalization. If the planned treatment is strictly elective, the physician will usually cancel the admission until the hospital's financial criteria have been met. At this point, assuming that the patient has no preexisting relationship with the hospital, the patient has no cause of action against the hospital's refusal of admission. However, the physician may have a cause of action against the hospital for interfering with the physician's practice, the damages being the fees lost through the hospital's refusal to admit the patient. If the admission is not strictly elective, the hospital's position is more precarious. The hospital administration cannot admit patients to the hospital; this privilege is limited to the members of the medical staff. While a veto by the administration over an admission is not exactly the same as an administrative decision to admit a patient, the result is the same: the administration has substituted its opinion for the physician's opinion. The legal question is whether anyone is injured by the veto. In the elective admission, the patient may suffer an injury by having the admission delayed. The physician's cause of action will still include the economic interest but will also include an action for indemnity if the hospital refusal of the patient causes the physician to be sued for malpractice.

If the physician classifies the admission as an emergency, the hospital is obliged to admit the patient. Refusing an emergency admission will result in almost certain liability if the patient is injured by the delay. This liability stems from the combination of the impermissible exercise of medical judgment by the administrator and the duty to render emergency care when the emergency is known and the physician has accepted the patient. The quality control manager must ensure that the admitting clerk does not turn away a patient without immediately informing the treating physician. The bylaws or section rules should provide a procedure for the physician to contest the refusal of admission, including the right to demand that the patient be admitted unless a medical reason is shown why the patient was refused admission and the time when the physician is able to have the patient admitted elsewhere.

Transfers

The transfer of a patient from one hospital to another, or from a hospital to a nursing home, is a medical decision that must be made by a physician. In this situation, the administrator may be able to argue that the patient's best interest requires a transfer to a different facility. The patient may need more specialized acute care than the hospital can render, or the patient may need the special skills of a chronic care facility. The administrator must be able to persuade the attending physician that the transfer is necessary to avoid injuring the patient. If the attending physician is unwilling to authorize the transfer, it may be necessary to persuade another member of the medical staff to arrange it. The medical section rules and hospital bylaws should have a procedure for such third party review of the need to transfer a patient.

The patient must be consulted about the transfer and informed of the reasons why it is necessary. A written consent should be obtained for the transfer and incorporated in the medical record. If the patient is unwilling to be transferred, legal complications may arise from transferring the patient against the patient's will. When the hospital admits the patient, it implicitly agrees to render care to the patient until the patient can be safely discharged. As noted earlier in the study on hospital liability, there may be situations where the patient poses a danger to others and thus may be transferred, after appropriate legal proceedings, to a more secure facility. The legal basis for transferring patients for their own good, as opposed to the safety of other patients, is not well-established. Since the law does not require all hospitals to offer the same level of technical expertise, there is a legal duty to recommend and facilitate a patient's transfer if this is necessary for the patient's well-being. However, the patient retains the right, after being given proper information, to choose not to be transferred. The hospital should honor the patient's decision to refuse a transfer, but this refusal should be put in writing, including detailed reasons for the request to transfer and the risks of refusing transfer.

The hospital must be careful not to overstate the benefits of a transfer. A common problem involves the transfer to a city or county hospital. It is very common for patients to be told that their care will be free at the county hospital. In most states this is true only if the patient meets both locality and income eligibility requirements. Most transfer patients will not meet these criteria and will be charged for their care, often at private hospital rates. The hospital must also ensure that the proposed facility can actually render the necessary care and that it has room for the patient. The only way to ensure this is to call ahead before transferring the patient.

False Imprisonment

If the hospital does not want to honor the patient's decision to refuse a transfer, the hospital should request a judicial ruling on the issue. Failure to obtain such an order could subject the health care provider to liability for false imprisonment. False imprisonment is the tort of restraining a person that person's will. The person may be physically restrained (tied up or locked up), restrained by drugs, or restrained by threats. The person does not need to try to escape. The recovery in a lawsuit based on false imprisonment includes damages for physical harm and psychological harm. False imprisonment is not based on negligence; it is an "intentional" tort, in that it is based on the "intent" to confine the person. This means that there is no community standard defense for false imprisonment. All competent adults (except for prisoners, soldiers, and so on) are legally entitled to be physically free in their movements. There is no special exception that allows hospital patients to be held against their will.

They do not have the right to interfere with the care of other patients, but they cannot be held in the hospital against their will. The problem of false imprisonment usually arises in the context of patients who want to leave the hospital before they are formally discharged. All competent adults have the right to leave the hospital at their own discretion. This right also allows parents or guardians to remove minor children from the hospital. The hospital has a duty to warn a patient of the risks entailed in leaving before it is medically indicated, but it does not have the right to restrain the patient. The hospital should inform the patient's admitting physician as soon as possible. The physician may be able to persuade the patient to stay, thus obviating the problem.

IMPLEMENTATION PROJECTS

Many computerisation projects have been undertaken in New Jersey and across the nation to attempt to improve the quality of healthcare and reduce the cost of healthcare administration. In this section we will describe several projects which the HINT team has studied that have the potential to reduce healthcare costs in New Jersey. For discussion purposes, the projects have been divided into three categories: projects ongoing within New Jersey, projects ongoing in other states, and projects which if undertaken within New Jersey could have significant quality and cost benefits.

Ongoing Projects within New Jersey

The HINT team's field research identified the following computerisation projects in various stages of development that have potential for delivering significant cost savings.

New Jersey Uniform Billing Committee

The Healthcare Finance Administration (HCFA) set up the National Uniform Billing Committee (NUBC) to establish a standard for the submission of Medicaid Claims as Uniform Billing—92 (UB-92). As part of this mandate, each state was urged to establish a State Uniform Billing Committee (SUBC) to provide specifications for reporting state specific data in "unlabeled fields designated for state use [UB-92 Data Element Specifications, 1993]. The original specifications were dated January 8, 1993. The specifications had an initial implementation date of October 1, 1993 with a three month window (ending December 31, 1993) where either the old from (UB-82) or the new form (UB-92) could be used. After December 31, 1993 the UB-82 form could no longer be used.

Accordingly, the New Jersey Uniform Billing Committee was establish in early 1993, chaired by the Department of Health (DOH) and comprised of consultants from the information technology industry, representatives from hospitals and representatives from insurance carriers. The committee recently (November 16, 1993) successfully defined how the "unlabeled state specific fields" would be used for hospital billing transactions within New Jersey.

NJ Specific Instructions

The "Uniform Billing Data Element Specifications, Modified for use in New Jersey" contain more that 50 pages of detailed instructions on the use of the "unlabeled state specific fields" [NJUBC, 1993]. By way of example the first two pages of general instructions are included below.

General Instructions for New Jersy UB-92

Only those data elements listed on the tape submission format, included as Appendix A, are required by the Department of Health. Each of these elements can be obtained or calculated from information contained on the UB-92 billing form. Beginning with discharges from January 1, 1994 forward, the Department of Health will no longer require or accept zero-filled ICD-9-CM codes.

All codes must be left-justified in their appropriate field locations. Nine (9) diagnosis and eight (8) procedure codes will continue to be required. Only inpatient and same day surgery outpatient discharge data need be submitted to the Department of Health. Replacement pages have been provided for those UB-92 data elements with unique requirements for New Jersey. Please put these in your manual at the appropriate place. The New Jersey Physician License Number will continue to be required for all discharges submitted to the Department of Health. This will be in addition to the billing requirement for the Uniform Physician Identification Number (). This License Number is now a 12 position field and will accept out-of-state codes for both Attending or Other Physicians. Please precede these License Numbers with their State Code.

NAC mapping for inappropriate use of certain General Classifications codes in ancillary services will no longer occur. This is reflected in Appendix B, Revenue Code Mapping to UB-92 Table Elements. Regardless of the financial fiscal year for hospitals required to submit data under N.J.A.C. 8:31B-2, all data will now be collected by calendar year. Beginning with discharges from January 1, 1994 forward, the data intermediary will be instructed to release to the Department of Health all first quarter 1994 records on June 30, 1994. The current requirement for the Department of Health to receive the UB-92 data within 90 days of the end of each calendar quarter will now apply to all hospitals.

Only specific bill types will be accepted by the Department of Health. Patient Status "22" & "23" have been deleted from use for patients discharged from New Jersey hospitals. These codes were developed for New York hospitals, not the New York Grouper.

The reporting of routine codes under UB-92 requires separate reporting of room charges with different rates even if their revenue codes are the same.

In order to report birth weight on a hard copy UB-92, please use Value Code 80.

Blood reporting has been moved to Value Codes 37, 38 and 39.

Payer Deductibles (A1, B1, C1), Coinsurance Amounts (A2, B2, C2), and Estimated Responsibility Amounts (A3, B3, C3, D3) are now Value Codes as indicated.

The patient's birthday now includes the full year designation, eliminating the need to collect a century indicator.

The patient's marital status, Form Locator 16, will now be collected.

Condition Codes, Occurrence Codes and Dates, and Value Codes have been assigned for Injury Prevention

Reporting requirements. Accident information should still be reported in addition to the specific codes assigned for Injury Prevention Reporting.

Medical Record Number now has its own location in Form Locator 23.

Due to the elimination of specific locations on the UB-92 to collect charges for each payer, the Department of Health will no longer require collection of this data. Appendix A, the tape submission format, reflects this change.

In order to accommodate long length of stay patients, the days reported in Form Locator 2 have been expanded to 4 bytes each. Additionally, transfer in/out facility codes have been moved to Value Codes 83 & 84, Form Locators 39-41.

In an effort to improve the reliability of UB-92 data to be used to develop Quality Indicators, Condition Code 82: Do Not Resuscitate Order on File, and Value Codes 81: Mother's Medical Record, and 82: Baby 5 minute Apgar Score, have been added to the data collection requirements.

For Medicaid only, Condition Code 80: Claim for Medicare Deductible or Coinsurance, and Value Code X9: New York DRG Rate, have been added to the billing form. Please refer to your Medicaid instructions for use of these codes.

In order to report a patient readmitted within 7 days of a previous acute care hospitalisation, please use Condition Code 81.

The detail described in these twenty two instructions is very specific and represents agreement among many of the healthcare industry specialists who are involved with the every day implementation of electronic data entry, storage and transmission. Many compromises were made to reach agreement but all participants accepted and implemented these standards. It should be noted that implementation does not require supplier specific hardware or software.

The HCFA and the New Jersey UB-92 is an example of a de jure standard with detailed specifications developed by joint decision of representatives from all parts of a heterogeneous industry. Historically, most detailed implementations of standards have been accomplished with defacto standards developed by powerful suppliers of information technology. But, defacto standards invariably benefit one technology supplier over others and therefore fail to receive widespread acceptance by users who have other supplier specific technology already installed. In other words, de facto standards tend to become proprietary standards rather than universal standards. The UB-92 standards are truly universal and, as such, are free of supplier favouritism.

New Jersey Electronic Birth Certificate

The New Jersey Electronic Birth Certificate (EBC) Project utilizes computers to increase programme and fiscal accountability in programme design, evaluation, quality assurance, and routine data processing in perinatal health. Specifically, this project was developed by the New Jersey Hospital Association's research and development arm, the Health Research and Educational Trust (HRET), to fully computerize creation, transmission, compilation, and distribution of birth certificate information. When fully operational in 1995, this system will allow hospital personnel to enter birth information on a computer and generate paper copies of the birth certificate while electronically transmitting the legal and confidential medical information about the birth for automatic inclusion in the state's computerized database. Whereas today, multiply redundant forms are filled out at the hospital and sent to various divisions in Trenton. The utility of an EBC system is well documented. Versions of an electronic birth certificate exist throughout most of the country. However, these other systems often rely on the exchange of floppy disks and focus more narrowly on the birth certificate. New Jersey's EBC was developed to serve as the data repository for a broader perinatal information network and will replace all existing paper-based reporting of duplicate information to the Departments of Heath and Human Services.

To date, the technology used in New Jersey to gather information and produce the birth certificate has been antiquated; indeed, the last technological advance to be applied to this process was the introduction of carbon paper. Currently, hospital staff spend considerable time collecting information (5 hours), typing (1 hour) and manually correcting (or retyping, as necessary for a legal document with multiple carbons) just to complete the birth certificate form. Time spent on these clerical duties represents time spent away from patient care and instructional activities or additional money spent on clerical assistance. And the hospital literature clearly identifies paperwork as a major point of hospital employee dissatisfaction [HRET, 1993].

Computerisation will significantly reduce data input time and enhance accuracy because editing will be done at the hospital through the software before the paper certificates are printed. The certificate will be printed on a laser printer at the hospital, signatures of the parents affixed and the completed paper original will be sent to the local registrar to be forwarded onto the State for archival purposes. The data in the completed EBC will be sent by modem directly to the state Department of Health. Data collected previously at the hospital, such as names, addresses and insurance information, can be automatically imported from the hospital's information system through a connection to the EBC local area network. The software will accept an electronic signature from the birth attendant and has been specifically designed to ease physician compliance yet protect patient and physician confidentiality.

Project Goal

The goal of the HRET project has been stated as: To develop and implement an information system to provide electronic transmission of state-mandated perinatal data. This project will provide more complete, accurate, and timely information through an information management solution that decreases the amount of data entry and processing work both by the hospital and the state.

Project Objectives

Six objectives have been identified:

1. To enable hospitals to automate the production of state-mandated perinatal data, including birth certificates, maternity and newborn logs, newborn hearing screening forms and the new certificate of parentage, with on-site (hospital) edits.
2. To create a system that will enable the electronic transmission of birth certificates to the Bureau of Vital Statistics.
3. To train designated hospital staff to use the programme and provide on-going support and training to hospitals.
4. To develop a set of uniform definitions and suggested data collection and entry procedures to increase the reliability and validity of perinatal data and promote the efficiency of its collection.
5. To develop an electronic mail or bulletin board capability between hospital maternity units and

between the hospitals and the state for the transmission of information, research, and updating the database.

6. To develop a set of reports within the perinatal database to provide hospitals with Joint Commission indicator requirements as well as support ad hoc quality assurance activities.

The proposed system would eliminate most of the data entry at the Bureau of Vital Statistics and provide information for data analysis and quality assurance. Department of Health data quality edits will be built into the data entry system at the hospital level. Currently, errors caught on computer edits at the state level are sent back to the hospital causing extensive searches through archived hospital records for patients discharged months before. This wastes scarce and expensive medical record staff time at the hospital. In addition to the increased quality of the data, the proposed system will allow health services managers and professionals at the New Jersey Department of Health's Center for Health Statistics and the Division of Maternal and Child Health flexibility for data analysis using inexpensive, commercially available statistical programmes (EPIINFO, PC SAS, dBASE, LOTUS, etc.) within the constraints of confidentiality and the data elements being collected.

Tasks

The project was broken down into nine tasks.

Task 1: Advisory Board: HRET established an Advisory Board consisting of experts in perinatal health from the Maternal And Child Consortia, data systems experts, and representatives from hospital maternity programmes, the Department of Health, including the Bureau of Vital Statistics, Center for Health Statistics, MMIS, Maternal and Child Health Services. The Board met at regular intervals to select software and now meets on an as needed basis.

Task 2: Contract for Computer Software System: The project management team identified software programmes and necessary changes to meet electronic birth certificate and maternity report requirements. HRET negotiated the customisation of the software and a long term licensing agreement with a competitively selected software vendor. The license will be held by the New Jersey Department of Health.

Task 3: Modify System Package: Management sought and incorporated feedback from medical records departments and maternity managers on the programme and pilot training sessions. Additionally, hardware requirements were determined and capability assessed at participating hospitals. Discount hardware packages will be offered to hospitals through New Jersey Hospital Association's Group Purchasing Programme, and statewide training sessions begin December 1, 1994.

Task 4: Concurrent Evaluation of Current System: HRET carried out an evaluation of the paper based birth certificate system to establish a baseline of time and cost prior to trials of the computer based system. A separate evaluation is being conducted by the School of Public Health at University of Medicine and Dentistry of New Jersey in Piscataway.

Task 5: Develop Database: HRET and the New Jersey Department of Health staffs have developed a data dictionary and customized database (New Jersey specific fields). Sample Electronic and paper reports have been sent to the Department of Health for feedback.

Task 6: Modify Database: The database will be modified as needed. Given the generic nature of the data base structure, such modifications will not be difficult. Record additions to the database will continue through this period. Additional output forms will be created as necessary.

Task 7: System Maintenance: Continue to run the system and perform debugging routines. Test at four hospitals with follow up training and trouble-shooting at the hospitals. The Advisory Board will meet quarterly to review the system and the quality of data. Staff will work with hospitals to facilitate electronic transfer of vital record data. The expected roll out date for all hospitals is January 1, 1995.

Task 8: Training Sessions: Over a six month period, the New Jersey Hospital Association Division UP Plus will conduct training sessions for clusters of hospitals utilizing software support staff for technical backup as needed.

Task 9: Evaluation: Evaluation of system performance will be conducted in a number of hospitals and at the Department of Health. The evaluation component of the project will be conducted by the Health Research and Educational Trust, headed by the Director of the Office of Health Policy Analysis. As a minimum, the following questions will be considered:

— Do hospital staff use the system?

— Does the hospital staff like it?

— Do the patients like it?

— Does it save time and money (nursing vs. clerical; collecting and entering information, typing, etc.)?

— Do hospital staff use the system for internal quality improvement reports?

— Do hospital staff use the system to communicate with other institutions, HRET, or the NJDOH?

— Does the system save NJDOH time and money?

— Is there any difference in the kind and amount of

analysis done at NJDOH since the advent of the system?

— Is the system cost effective?

A set of quantitative measures will be developed during the project trial period to better assess the value of the project and support the qualitative measures above.

Summary of the Birth Records Project

This project was set up to solve a paper logjam in hospitals—birth certificate preparation and recording. By converting to an electronic data entry, transmission and storage system, the project management team created a win-win situation where the hospitals solved a problem, realised reduced costs and created a database for clinical quality improvement projects. Manual data entry of birth records at the state will be discontinued thereby saving the state money and assuring more accuracy and timeliness of the records. Birth records will be stored in a easily accessible electronic data base that researchers and other users can access with the analytical software of their choice. The next project, the NJ Comprehensive Immunisation Programme, benefits directly from the establishment of the electronic birth record system.

New Jersey Comprehensive Immunisation Programme (NJ-CIP)

Children can be immunized against most serious childhood diseases rather easily and at little or no cost to their parents. The problem is that these diseases are so rarely encountered in society today, that parents consider the immunisation process an unnecessary bother. Yet, periodically, epidemics of these diseases break out, even among young adults where they present more serious health risks. For example, a measles epidemic broke out among Rutgers University students in the spring of 1994. The question is, "What can the state do to encourage parents to have their children immunized at the proper age?" An important answer emerged when the Robert Wood Johnson Foundation awarded a one year planning grant, "New Jersey Immunisation Improvement Project", to Principal Investigator David H. Carver, MD, Professor and Chairman of Pediatrics, Robert Wood Johnson Medical School, University of Medicine and Dentistry of New Jersey. Dr. Carver and CO-Principal Investigator Dr. Kenneth Spitalny (State Epidemiologist, NJDOH) were subsequently awarded a three year implementation grant by the Robert Wood Johnson Foundation for the design, pilot testing and implementation of an immunisation registry for New Jersey preschool children.

The implementation grant, running from August 1, 1993 through July 31, 1996, is titled "New Jersey Comprehensive Immunisation Program" (NJ-CIP). The grant integrates activities to be carried out by the project's collaborators, who are:

— University of Medicine and Dentistry of New Jersey, Robert Wood Johnson Medical School, Department of Pediatrics;
— NJ Department of Health (Commissioner's Office, WIC Programme and Immunisation Program);
— NJ Department of Human Services (Commissioner's Office, and AFDC Program);
— NJ Chapter of the American Academy of Pediatrics;
— Computer consultants (Rutgers University, and University of Pennsylvania);
— Health economists (Wharton School, University of Pennsylvania);
— Community based healthcare providers; and

— Community based health educators.

NJ-CIP Goal

The major goal of the NJ-CIP is to create a New Jersey computerized preschool immunisation registry and outreach system, in order to improve immunisation coverage rates. Currently, a registry and outreach pilot project is under way in Camden, New Jersey. The pilot project initially is targeting Aid to Families with Dependent Children (AFDC) and Women with Infants and Children (WIC) preschoolers, and will phase in preschool children in Camden who receive their healthcare in hospital clinics, other public clinics, and the offices of private physicians. The pilot project will attempt to link each Camden child lacking a regular source of medical care with a comprehensive healthcare provider. And then encourage the parent(s) to have the child immunized. The Leonard Davis Institute of Health Economics (LDI) of the University of Pennsylvania will evaluate the effectiveness and cost efficiency of the Registry and other interventions in improving the immunisation status of NJ preschool children.

Statewide Implementation

The Project will subsequently be replicated at additional sites in the state. The NJ-CIP also is actively designing immunisation education materials and presentations for professionals (both physicians and nurses) and the lay public.

Interface to the National Registry

The concept is to design a Registry database with both data collection and query (front-end) and data repository (back-end) capability with consistent user interfaces and standard file transfer protocol and applications to be deployed in all settings. The back-end, front-end concept corresponds to the Center for Disease Control (CDC) National Immunisation Programme (NIP) design specifications thus assuring that NJ will be able to participate in Interstate and State-to-CDC communications. Although the initial NJ-CIP Registry is provider-based, its intention is to utilize birth records and the Hepatitis B immunisation (in most cases, administered in the hospital at birth) as an initializing record in the Registry.

The Registry design incorporates birth record and Hepatitis B immunisation data from the Electronic Birth Certificate described in section 4.1.2 New Jersey Electronic Birth Certificate above. The Registry data model and data elements have been developed in conjunction with the record layout for the EBC, and Health Research and Education Trust (HRET) has included these in the EBC data dictionary. The implementation of the EBC in January 1995 will make possible the timely availability of birth demographics and the initial Hepatitis B immunisation for inclusion in the Registry.

Access to the State Registry

Access to the registry will be Internet based, thereby leveraging existing infrastructure and incorporating standard open system, EDI communication standards. This assures the registry and immunisation communications will support both intra-State and inter-state initiatives. Providers will access the network via high speed dial-up (for small sites) or Integrated Services Data Network (ISDN) (for larger sites). The project will build, maintain, and support Internet based information about the Project and immunisations in general. This includes providing and operating Internet-based servers (such as Gopher and World-Wide Web) containing information about the project as well as pointers to other information of interest to the target audience.

Immunisation Project Summary

This is an example of a major new initiative to improve

overall community health that is possible primarily because of the application of computer technology to:

- Identify target citizens,
- Direct and guide citizens to the required medical services
- Measure actual service delivery, and
- Maintain a service delivery data base to assess project effectiveness.

The core of this project is the use of standard data entry, storage, communication, application, and transmission protocols. The communication system is an existing open system, available to all who choose to connect. The benefits will be realised with minimal cost because the programme uses available technologies and builds upon existing computerized record systems (birth records). This is a model EDI application that promises to improve the quality of life for New Jersey citizens.

Lauri Imaging Center MRI—EDI Link

The Lauri Imaging Center in New Brunswick, part of the Robert Wood Johnson Hospital, has developed a pilot remote access system to retrieve radiological records, including the full images and doctors' notes, using the Mosaic Presentation Software on Workstations, PCs and MACs. This is an important example of improved services through the use of available, low cost technology. First, we will explain what Mosaic is and Mosaic's power as a presentation system. Subsequently, we will discuss how the Lauri Imaging Center uses Mosaic as an EDI system for MRI distribution.

Mosaic Presentation Software

Before continuing with the discussion of radiology image transmission and describing the Lauri Image transmission system, it is useful to describe the Mosaic presentation system that Lauri Imaging uses. After this brief digression, we will return to describing Lauri Image's system. The Mosaic presentation system, a recent development of the National Center for Supercomputer Applications (NCSA) at the University of Illinois, is based on the World Wide Web (WWW) developed at CERN in Switzerland with extensions based on the EIES software developed by NJIT.

The user simply uses a mouse to select a document and the text and any accompanying images are delivered to the Mosaic window. While the user reads the text the images are loaded. Each image has a distinctive file extension which denotes the viewing/listening software that is evoked to display/play the image. Once loaded, the images can be viewed by clicking a mouse on the icon representing each image. The appropriate software is automatically evoked.

Mosaic requires either direct access to a network via a Transmission Control Protocol/Internet Protocol (TCP/IP) package and/or modem access using a Serial Line Interface Protocol (SLIP) or Point-to-Point Protocol (PPP). Mosaic software is available free on the Internet from NCSA via anonymous File Transfer Protocol (FTP). Mosaic requires Microsoft Windows 32 bit extensions for use on a PC with Windows 3.1, available free from Microsoft over the Internet via anonymous FTP. Point to Point Protocol is a reasonably priced commercial package. Trumpet, a shareware version of SLIP, is available free for trials and may be obtained for continued use for a nominal fee.

Four features of the Mosaic interface make it ideal for viewing documents on-line:

> Mosaic utilizes a system of screen formatting called Hyper Text Markup Language (HTML). HTML allows individuals creating documents to

imbed formatting notations (markups) in the body of the text. These notations are converted to formatting commands when the document is displayed using Mosaic. For example, <b> imbedded in the text selects a bold font, </b> restores the normal font and <p> inserts a paragraph break. Using this notation the writer can create on-line documents that are nearly identical to printed text making reading of the document much easier. In, addition, the reader can scroll up and down through the document at will to reread any paragraph.

If the reader would like a copy of the document saved on a local disk drive, Mosaic has a 'load to disk' option which once selected will cause all file requests to be saved to the local drive instead of displayed. To facilitate the process even further, Mosaic has a 'reload button', which when depressed (a mouse click), will request the file a second time—i.e. for saving on the local drive. Mosaic incorporates multimedia capabilities. Image, audio and video objects can be imbedded in the HTML text through references similar to the bold font <b> described above. Each type of object has a file extension which causes Mosaic to invoke the appropriate player or viewer. For example, the extension "gif" displays graphic images. The character string <img src="file:///c:njit.gif"> imbedded in a HTML document located on a NJIT computer will display the NJIT logo as part of the document.

Mosaic allows authors to link documents to other objects by the use of anchors. The anchor is imbedded in the text as a reference similar to the graphic image above. The anchor could be used as a footnote or reference to the text. The anchor could also display an abstract of a document with a further anchor in the abstract to the entire document or to the entire document's table of contents. For example, if the following sentence (with the imbedded character string):

> HL7 standards are available at
>
> <ahref="http:://dumccss.mc.duke.edu/ftp/standards.html">DUKE</a> University.
>
> was included in a document, the text would be displayed as:
>
> HL7 standards are available at DUKE University.

The word 'DUKE' appears with the text and is underscored and in color (usually blue). The underscore and the color denotes that the word or phrase is an 'anchor' to another object (document, graphic, video, sound bite, etc.). Using a mouse and 'clicking' on the underscored word causes Mosaic to request the object via the Internet. There is no limit to the number of anchors in a document or the number of succeeding documents that can be accessed via anchors. The Mosaic technology allows specific images to be imbedded into the text much like a book where tables and/or charts appear adjacent to text relevant to their content. Mosaic, therefore facilitates the readers' understanding of the text by providing images with specific reference positions in the text. For highly technical documents, such as a radiologist's evaluation of an MRI, Mosaic provides an ideal retrieval and display system.

Lauri Imaging MRI—EDI System Operation

In the current method of examination, when a patient undergoes a MRI, the radiologist monitors the progress using the MRI equipment video screen, adding sections as necessary to conduct a full diagnostic evaluation. When the MRI is complete, the digital output is converted to a film recording. The radiologist reads the film and writes up or dictates the appropriate diagnosis. The diagnosis is sometimes discussed with the patient. However in almost all cases the film and the diagnosis (radiologist's notes) are forwarded to the requesting physician. Because most physicians practice in various locations, MRI diagnoses may not reach the requesting physician in a timely manner. However, if the diagnosis and images are loaded onto a computer at the radiologist's office, EDI access to the MRI data can occur within minutes after the radiologist completes the diagnosis.

Working with its MRI equipment vendor, the Lauri Imaging Center was able to develop translation routines that convert MRI images into a Mosaic presentation format. Each individual MRI image is translated into a separate file. The files are saved in a '.gif' format for direct viewing using Mosaic. A medical secretary transcribes the diagnosis into a document formatted as a HTML file. During the transcription process, the secretary creates the anchors for the appropriate MRI images, using the file names included as part of the dictation. Once the transcription is complete, the files are placed in password protected location on a computer file server. A mail message or telephone call alerts the requesting physician to the availability of the MRI information. The physician logs into the file server using the Mosaic software and reads the diagnosis. While the text is being read, small copies of the MRI images (icons) are brought up as part of the diagnosis document. When the physician is ready to view a full MRI image, a mouse 'click' on the icon brings it to the screen. Back and forth arrow buttons on the Mosaic toolbar allow the physician to switch between the text and each of the images.

Radiology via an EDI Network

The Lauri Center's MRI—EDI project demonstrates that radiological images can be transmitted effectively using commercially available software and an existing commercial

EDI network or dial up telephone lines. Thus, it is reasonable to assume that in the near future EDI systems established for administrative data transfer will eventually be equally useful to transfer even the most complex of medical data—radiological images.

NJIT Model for a Medical Office Workstation

Although nearly all group practices have practice management systems; most individual providers do not utilize computers to manage their practices. Even among the groups and individual practitioners who do have computers, however, few utilize electronic claims transactions. Furthermore, the majority of physicians do not have computer access to clinical records outside their office. Nurses' notes, laboratory test results, etc. are, at best, transmitted by FAX rather than available through computerized physician inquiry.

It should be noted that computer communication among providers is a moot subject until the majority of physicians have computers in their offices for practice management. A EDI system with only five or ten percent of the providers connected is a useless system. Since it is probable that hardware and software costs may be a factor in physicians' decisions on whether to use computers, NJIT decided to develop a pilot demonstration of a low cost physician office practice system.

The primary project objective is to provide the physician a system that would yield the major cost savings benefits of EDI administrative transactions while involving the minimum investment in hardware and software. If such an inexpensive system was available, more physicians may choose to join the computer/EDI system. In addition, if the same system could be used to access laboratory reports and view radiological images, even more providers would find it useful. Therefore, the second objective of the project was to produce a workstation that would demonstrate EDI connectivity for radiological and other medical images. The project was broken down into four phases:

- Select appropriate platform with the appropriate software
- Develop a billing information management system
- Develop methods to send, receive, display and print billing information
- Develop methods to send, receive and display graphic images

Task 1. Select Appropriate Platform and Applications Software

The objective of phase one was to select a platform and applications software which were: inexpensive, readily obtainable, adequate for the envisioned tasks and yet expandable to meet future, as yet undetermined needs.

Platform: The IBM compatible PC was selected as the platform. Such machines are widely available, highly reliable, and very competitively priced. The minimum configuration for a provider was established to be:

- A 80486/SX25 processor with an over-drive socket for future expansion
- A desktop or mini-tower (desk top on end) case with 101 key keyboard
- Eight megabytes of main memory
- A 170 megabyte hard drive and single 3.5" 1.44 megabyte floppy drive
- A 14" super VGA monitor with a 1 megabyte video card (1024 x 768 resolution)
- A 14,400 baud internal fax-modem with FAX software

— A Microsoft compatible mouse

— MS-DOS operating system (Ver 6.22) and Microsoft windows (Ver 3.10)

The current street price for a national brand name IBM compatible PC in the above configuration is under $1,300 The configuration could be upgraded in speed by a factor of 3 to 1 by selecting a 80486/DX2-66 processor for $250 additional. If the provider's office required more than one PC, Microsoft Windows for Workgroups and an Ethernet card could be added to each PC for an additional $200.

Available (off the shelf) Software: Unquestionably, off the shelf commercial software is the least expensive way to equip such a machine. Custom designed software costs five to twenty times as much as off the shelf. The Microsoft Office package (Ver 4.2) was selected as the base-line software configuration. The package has a street price of about $280. The package includes:

— Microsoft Word (Ver 6.0a)—word processor

— Microsoft Excel (Ver 5.0)—spread sheet

— Microsoft Power Point (Ver 4.0)—presentation software

— Microsoft Mail—advanced E-mail tools

As an add-on, the Microsoft Office Assistant package was selected. This package has a street price of $65. The package includes:

— Microsoft Office Assistant—Business management tools and forms

— Microsoft Access (Ver 2.0)—database management software

The total cost for the hardware and software for the

provider's office is $1,650. This configuration provides all of the standard software to run a small office and dial-in to remote points to access information from other sources. Other popular software packages are available at similar prices.

Development Software: Microsoft Visual Basic Professional (Ver 3.0) was selected as a development tool. It has a street price of $300. Visual Basic will only be used by developers and is not required in the providers office. Visual Basic enables a developer to create custom applications using the software on the provider's PC with direct linkage into:

— The WORD word processor for transcribing notes, creating referral letters, etc.

— The EXCEL spread sheet for calculating costs, preparing purchase orders and invoices, etc.

— The ACCESS database for entering information into the office or patient databases

— The Windows Terminal Emulator for connecting to remote sites

— The Windows Calendar for scheduling appointments

— The Windows Calculator for quick math

When Visual Basic is used to control these applications, the developer can create an integrated solution which acts as a alternate to the normal access to each individual applications. This solution offers a custom tailored suite of functions for the administration of a provider's office.

Task 2. Develop a Solution to Manage Billing Information

Currently, many physicians with individual practices do not file claims for their patients. However, this is rapidly changing as managed care begins to dominate among the alternative health benefit plans. Thus, it is probable that most, perhaps all physicians, will be sending claims or patient visit (encounter) reports directly to payers in the near future. Therefore, the primary administrative system required for a physician computerized practice system is a billing/claim filing system.

Create a Billing Database—Build a HCFA 1500 Data Entry Screen: The first problem encountered in creating a provider's billing database was to determine what information had to be maintained in the database to provide adequate billing information. This was complicated by the fact that there are over 450 medical claim forms in use in the United States. Selecting an appropriate claim form for use in New Jersey proved easier that expected.

The Healthcare Financing Administration (HCFA) published a revised set of standard forms in 1992 under the title Uniform Billing 1992 (UB92). These forms, HCFA 1450 for providers and HCFA 1500 for hospitals, are the mandatory forms for submission of Medicare claims beginning in 1994. Since each state administers Medicaid locally, the New Jersey Department of Human Services, the state's Medicaid agency, convened the New Jersey Uniform Billing Committee to plan an implementation schedule for the new form for Medicaid within the state. The committee planned on implementation of the new forms beginning in October 1993. Therefore, it seemed logical to use the HCFA 1450 form as the basis for a data entry screen for physicians. In addition, work is in progress to convert the present flat file electronic submission format of the HCFA 1450 and 1500 forms into an electronic standard X12 format as described in Section 3.3.7 "Transaction 837—Healthcare Claim."

The HCFA 1450 contains all of the data blocks necessary for the claim. All of this data, with the exception of the specific visit information, if captured once, can be used over and over. Therefore, a simple database was designed to maintain patient records and file claims while eliminating redundant data entries. The data was broken down as follows: facility information, provider information, patient information, benefit information, payer information, nomenclature tables, visit information and claim (adjudication) information.

Facility Information: The legal entity, federal and state tax IDs, street address, mailing address, telephone and fax numbers, contact name.

Provider Information: Providers name, local ID, profession, federal and state licenses, SSN.

Patient Information: Name, ID(SSN), address, telephone number, age, sex, marital status, next of kin, and emergency number (Other information such as occupation, employer, race, height, weight, allergies and medical history could be included, but are not necessary for billing information). Benefits Information: Patient ID, Carrier ID, policy number (group, coverage, etc.), subscriber, relationship to subscriber, deductibles, co-pay, etc.

Carrier Information: Carrier Name, ID, address, telephone number, fax number, contact person.

Nomenclature Tables: Initial Classification of Disease (ICD-9) and Current Procedural Terminology (CPT-4) tables to match codes to the descriptions and a billing table for individual and grouped procedures (A cross reference table of ICD versus appropriate CPT could be added).

Visit Information: Local claim number, carrier claim number, patient ID, provider ID, date, line number, ICD, CPT and charges.

Claim Information: Local claim number, carrier claim number, line number, allowable charges(capitation), deductible, co-payment, net amount.

Task 3. Develop Methods to Send, Receive, Display and Print Billing Information

The display and printing of the visit, claim and adjudication data could be done on one page with a laser printer. Using the Visual Basic Language, the page could be made to look like the HCFA 1450. However, if real-time electronic submission was used, then the only printed output will be a receipt to the patient. This could be inexpensively produced by standard credit card receipt printer with two part paper. This receipt could be produced to indicate in detail the claim numbers, patient name and ID, date, International Classification of Disease (ICD-9-CM) and Current Procedural Terminology (CPT-4) and the method of payment by the patient of those expenses exceeding the insurance reimbursement—i.e. cash, check or credit card. If a credit card payment, it would also serve as the credit card receipt. In either case the patient's signature on the receipt would authenticate the visit for any post visit audit. Sending the claim and receiving the adjudication was based on transactions in an ANS X12 837 format. This format is designed to serve as the electronic submission for both the HCFA 1450 and 1500 forms. The transaction is identified by it's number—837—in the initial data sequence. It uses the Group Separator (GS = ASCII 029) as the data element (field) separator <gs>, the File Separator (FS = ASCII 028) as the Segment Terminator <tr> and the Unit Separator (US = ASCII 126) as the subelement separator<us>. Blank elements are indicated by two or more adjacent group separators <gs>.

A File Separator is used to indicate the end of a segment and eliminates a series of <gs> if the remainder of the elements are blank or unused. Since there are special codes (unprintable characters), we included in the transaction software a conversion routine so that the transaction may be printed on any printer using the ASCII character set and is easily understood by anyone familiar with the transaction. We substituted asterisk (* = ASCII 042), Tilde (~ = ASCII 126) and the Carriage Return (<cr> = ASCII 013) for the <gs>, <us> and <tr> respectively. We assume that payers will have developed their computer systems to receive electronic claims transfer directly from providers, initially on tape and then via direct transmission and that an open EDI system can be made available to support this technology. The NJIT researchers used this software package to successfully develop the claims data base and screens for data entry and transmission of the 837 transaction set thereby demonstrating that this is a realistic low cost solution.

On August 29, 1993, the software was demonstrated to members of the New Jersey legislature and their staffs. Completion of the overall package can be inexpensively done by one or more commercial software firms in New Jersey. NJIT's initial work is available to any firms that are interested.

Task 4. Investigate Methods to Send, Receive and Display Radiology Images

There have been many discussions about ways to enable remote access to medical images such as X-rays and MRIs. The Lauri Imaging Center in New Brunswick, part of the Robert Wood Johnson Hospital, has piloted a system (Lauri Imaging Center MRI—EDI Link) to provide remote retrieval of MRI records, including the accompanying doctors notes and the full MRI images. Their work showed that MRI (digital) information could be transmitted and displayed on PC, MAC or X-window based workstations.

Perception: In the human eye the primary image receptor area contains approximately 340,000 image elements (cones) comprised of about 600 x 600 receptors. [Gonzalez and Woods, 1992] Inexpensive solid state electronic image sensors, such as Charge Coupled Devices (CCDs) [Gonzalez and Woods, 1992, p. 24], are available today that provide three times this resolution [Texas Instruments, 1991]. This means that the ability of the human eye to resolve image details is within the capability of existing electronic image sensors. However, psychovisual aspects of human perception of images may be even more important. Examples of this are the non-uniform perception of intensity and the strong influence of contrast on the perceived quality of an image.

Resolution: Luminance (or luminance factor)—usually denoted by the symbol Y—is a standard psychophysical term representing the physical quantity corresponding to the sensation of lightness in a scene, not to be confused with the video voltage signal representative of luminance [Billmeyer and Saltzman, 1981]. For a given object with known reflectance, a specific illuminant, and a certain observer it is straightforward to calculate the value of luminance factor Y. The spectral composition of luminance comprises of about 11% power from the blue regions, 59% from green and 30% from red. Contrast ratio is defined as the ratio of luminance between the lightest and darkest elements of a scene. An image with high contrast ratio may be judged of superior quality (sharper) over another of measurably higher spatial resolution but lower contrast ratio. Thus contrast ratio is a major determinant of image quality.

The human perception of luminance is the perceived lightness. The sensation of lightness can distinguish luminance levels within about a two-decade range, i.e. the eye is able to resolve a luminance variation (dL) up to about 1/100 increment [Gonzalez and Woods, 1991, p. 34]. The luminance discrimination threshold depends on the individual subject and the dark adaptation of the eye during the test. Human vision adapts over a remarkably large range of light intensity levels—about seven decades of dynamic range in total [Billmeyer and Saltzman, 1981]. At each adaptation state the human eye can discern a dynamic range as high as 100:1.

Experimental tests have been performed to determine the contrast sensitivity of human vision. In these tests most of the observer's field of vision is filled by a surround luminance level, L0, in order to fix the observer's state of adaptation. The tests have shown that there exists a range of more than two decades of luminance over which the discrimination capability of human vision is about 1% of the test luminance level. If codes, representing luminance steps, are placed at exactly 1% intervals over a 100:1 range, the number of codes required is log 100 / log 1.01, or 460 codes [Poynton, 1993, pp. 1099—1108]. These measurements of contrast sensitivity at threshold lead to a logarithmic relationship. However, this logarithmic relationship does not extend well from thresholds to large luminance ratios. Over a wider range of luminance, the lightness sensation is computed approximately as the cube root of physical luminance. The relationship is

$$L^* = 116 \text{ reg. } 1/3 - 16 \text{ for } r > 0.01 \text{ where } r = Y/Yn$$

$$L^* = 903.29 \text{ reg. for } r < 0.01$$

where L^* is the CIE psychometric (or metric) lightness, Y is the luminance factor and Yn is the value of Y for the reference white [Judd and Wyszecki, 1975]. By convention Yn = 100. CIE refers to the International Commission on Illumination (Commission International de l'Eclairage). In practice, coding a luminance signal to a lightness value by the use of a power law with an exponent between 0.33 and 0.45 has been found to perform excellently perceptually.

Color Models and Computer Graphics: A color model is a specification of a subspace of a 3-D coordinate system in which each point represents a color. Examples are the RGB (red, green, blue) model used in practice primarily for color monitors and video cameras, the CMY (cyan, magenta, yellow) for printers, and the YIQ (Y for luminance video signal, I for in phase, and Q for quadrature chromatic components) for color video broadcast. There is also the HSI model (hue, saturation, chromaticity) used for color image manipulation [Texas Instruments, 1991].

The three colors Red, Green and Blue can be combined in any proportion to generate most of the other colors. These proportions, if treated like coordinates, make up the tip of a vector roaming the inside of a cube of side 1, the color cube. That is, values of Red, Green, and Blue are assumed to be in the range of 0 to 1. If we move along the Red, Green and Blue axes in equal steps, the resulting colors are shades of gray.

Along the main diagonal there are two important points, the origin where

0.0 Red + 0.0 Green + 0.0 Blue = Black

and the other end of the diagonal, where

1.0 Red + 1.0 Green + 1.0 Blue = White [Texas Instruments, 1991].

Color images in the RGB model consist of three independent frames, one each for red, green and blue, the three primary colors. These three images drive the three phosphor screens of a color monitor. Most color cameras also use the RGB model when acquiring digital images.

Computer Implementation of the Color Model: As mentioned above, the RGB model provides three color screens, one each for red, green and blue; which may be used to drive the phosphors of a color display. Physically, these signals are provided by three digital to analog (D/A) converters in color computer graphics cards that convert a palette color entry into corresponding analog voltage levels. Typically, each of these D/A converters uses 8 bits to represent each primary color, so each can reproduce a range of color from 00 Hex to FF Hex (0 to 255) for red, green, and blue; in other words, each pixel has 24 bits of color information. Thus, the card can reproduce 256 x 256 x 256 = 16,777,216 different colors. However, human vision can discriminate only a small fraction of less than 5% of these colors. Since gray is a combination of equal parts of Red, Blue and Green, the graphics card is capable of producing 256 levels (shades) of Gray from Black (0) to White (255). The output of the graphics card is connected to a cathode ray tube (CRT). The CRT accepts the RGB analog voltage outputs as well as synchronisation information, amplifies them, and drives the phosphor guns to produce the image. However, in a CRT the input voltage is related to the output light luminance intensity non-linearly [Kennel and Snider, 1993]. This relation originates in the electrostatic interaction between the cathode and the control grid of the current of the electron beam. It is best described by

$$\text{light intensity} = (\text{input voltage} + b)\ 2.5$$

where

b is the black error level [Poynton, 1993].

By contrast the phosphors themselves respond linearly until they approach saturation [DeMarsh, 1993]. The exponent of 2.5 in the non-linear relation above is called the gamma, and the process of compensating for its departure from 1.0 (linearity) gamma correction. In a video system gamma correction is applied at the camera for the dual purpose of precompensating the non-linearity of the display's CRT and for coding into a perceptually uniform space. In viewing images on a display screen, typically a dim surround is in the backdrop. In such viewing conditions it turns out to be perceptually best to "stretch" the contrast ratio of the reproduced image. In video, the "stretching" is accomplished by slightly under compensating for the CRT. In fully compensating at the camera the gamma correction would be 1.0/2.5, so that when multiplied by 2.5 it produces an overall system gamma of 1.0, i.e. a linear end-to-end response. However, in actuality, the compensation is 1.0/2.2 , so the overall system gamma is 1.13. This technique produces pictures that are sharp, and quite pleasing when viewed in typical dim surroundings [Poynton, 1993].

Another problem with CRTs is that they have a Gaussian pixel intensity distribution of the transition from pixel to pixel or line to line; this transition is not crisp but depends on the variance around the mean of the intensity distribution. Lastly, as the intensity of gray levels increase in CRTs, the pixel width also increases. Such problems can be alleviated by choosing a high quality CRT display.

Experimental transmission of X-ray Images: The most common and widely used medical images are MRIs, CAT Scans and X-rays. MRIs and CAT Scans are produced in digital form first. However, like X-rays they are often captured on film for permanent records. As discussed earlier, the management of X-ray data is the most challenging issue in dealing with radiological images.

X-ray images were captured using a broadcast quality television camera connected to a PC with an interface card—a *frame grabber*. The images were stored on the PC's hard drive. They were displayed on the PC's monitor, in this case a super VGA monitor with a resolution of 1024 x 768 pixels using several different display software packages running under Microsoft Windows. The nominal size of the image captured during the experiments was approximately 330,000 bytes (pixels). It was displayed in a 640 x 480 pixel window. We also used a CCD camera, grabbing images of 1024 x 1024 pixels. For the CCD image, a PC with a display resolution of 1280 x 1024 was required to display the full image .

The images were transmitted in a manner similar to an ANS X12 864 Text Message (E-mail) transaction. A modified 864 transaction set was constructed which was arbitrarily termed a 964 Image Transfer transaction set. We added a new segment after the MSG segment of Table 2 which we labeled IMG for Image. The new IMG segment consisted of three different data elements. The first element of the IMG segment is the image type code. For this element we chose to use the existing Product/Service ID Qualifier 235 element which is an ID code consisting of two alpha-numeric characters. We chose the code XR to represent X-rays and MR for MRIs. Both codes are unused in the present 235 code list. The code list for this element would have to be expanded to accommodate additional image definitions.

The second and third elements of the IMG segment are the Length of the Binary Data, element 784, and the Binary Data, element 785. These two elements are currently used only in the BIN segment. However, the BIN segment has no Qualifier and is only used in the Specifications / Technical Information 841 transaction set which contains numerous extraneous, yet mandatory, segments. The Length of the Binary Data element consists of up to 15 digits representing integer numbers from -99,999,999,999,999 to 999,999,999,999,999. The Binary Data element consists of a series of eight bit bytes (octets) ranging in value from 00000000 binary to 11111111 binary (00 to FF hexadecimal, 0 to 255 decimal). We assumed that these element pairs could be repeated 99 times, once for each image needed in the transaction set.

By reusing all of the segments from the Text Message transaction set we were able to provide all of the identification information required plus the radiologist's diagnostic report along with the images in one X12 transaction set. Since we were only demonstrating the technology, we did not attempt to pack the image data, which could have reduced the transmission time. [As a side note, while testing the transmission of this data set, we obtained a binary file containing 32 bit extensions to the windows operating system from Microsoft Corporation in Redmond, WA. The file contained more than 1,200,000 bytes of information. The transmission, including the time on a LAN and storing the file on the PC's hard disk, took slightly less than two minutes via the Internet in the middle of a weekday afternoon.]

We viewed the text file and images on a PC using Microsoft Notepad and Paintbrush (parts of Windows) and VIEW and Mosaic, free graphical programmes. (MRI images from the Lauri Imaging Center were also received and displayed using Mosaic on this same computer.) With further work, the software could be made available at a nominal cost to accelerate the adoption of electronic means for claim and clinical information transfer.

In the overall evaluation of existing technology, it is apparent that off the shelf software combined with on site programme modifications can be used to produce a low to moderate priced office practice system that will enable even a small provider's office to utilize an EDI service along with other, more sophisticated users. As the majority of providers acquire low cost office computers that deliver administrative cost savings, they will likely join the EDI system to achieve cost savings in electronic transfer of claims. Then, as the majority of providers link into the EDI system, it will become an effective and efficient system for all providers and payers. Undoubtedly, as providers become more accustomed to the use of a practice management system, the use of the EDI system will become more widespread. It is probable that additional services will be added to the system by various vendors—medical abstract services, for example on a fee for service basis.

In addition, if the healthcare EDI system(s) are connected to the Internet, all participants can obtain the most current information at no additional cost. Thus, the EDI system will not only save administrative costs for all participants but also will create opportunities for expanded medical services that will contribute to improved healthcare for the community.

EVIDENCE-BASED REVIEW METHODOLOGY

Definition and Scope

For this project the UCSF-Stanford Evidence-Based Practice Center (EPC) defined a *patient safety practice* as "a type of process or structure whose application reduces the probability of adverse events resulting from exposure to the healthcare system across a range of conditions or procedures." Examples of practices that meet this definition include computerized physician order entry, thromboembolism prophylaxis in hospitalized patients, strategies to reduce falls among hospitalized elders, and novel education strategies such as the application of "crew resource management" to train operating room staff. By contrast, practices that are disease-specific and/or directed at the underlying disease and its complications (e.g., use of aspirin or beta-blockers to treat acute myocardial infarction) rather than complications of medical care are not included as "patient safety practices."

In some cases, the distinction between patient safety and more general quality improvement strategies is difficult to discern. *Quality improvement practices* may also qualify as patient safety practices when the current level of quality is considered "unsafe," but standards to measure safety are often variable, difficult to quantify, and change over time. For example, what constitutes an "adequate" or "safe" level of accuracy in electrocardiogram or radiograph interpretation? Practices to improve performance to at least the "adequate" threshold may reasonably be considered safety practices because they decrease the number of diagnostic errors of omission. On the other hand, we considered practices whose main intent is to improve performance above this threshold to be quality improvement practices. An example of the latter might be the use of computer algorithms to improve the sensitivity of screening mammography.

We generally included practices that involved acute hospital care or care at the interface between inpatient and outpatient settings. This focus reflects the fact that the majority of the safety literature relates to acute care and the belief that systems changes may be more effectively achieved in the more controlled environment of the hospital. However, practices that might be applicable in settings in addition to the hospital were not excluded from consideration.

For example, the Compendium includes practices for preventing decubitus ulcers that could be applied in nursing homes as well as hospitals. The EPC team received input regarding the scope of the Compendium from the Agency for Healthcare Research and Quality (AHRQ), which commissioned the report. In addition, the EPC team participated in the public meeting of the National Quality Forum (NQF) Safe Practices Committee on January 26, 2001. The NQF was formed in 1999 by consumer, purchaser, provider, health plan, and health service research organisations to create a national strategy for quality improvement. Members of the Safe Practices Committee collaborated with the EPC team to develop the scope of work that would eventually become this Compendium.

Organisation by Domains

To facilitate identification and evaluation of potential patient safety practices, we divided the content for the project into different *domains*. Some cover "content areas" (e.g., adverse drug events, nosocomial infections, and complications of surgery). Other domains involve identification of practices within broad (primarily "non-medical") disciplines likely to contain promising approaches to improving patient safety (e.g., information technology, human factors research, organisational theory). The domains were derived from a general reading of the literature and were meant to be as inclusive as possible. The list underwent review for completeness by patient safety experts, clinician-researchers, AHRQ, and the NQF Safe Practices Committee. For each domain we selected a team of author/collaborators with expertise in the relevant subject matter and/or familiarity with the techniques of evidence-based review and technology appraisal. The authors, all of whom are affiliated with major academic centers around the United States.

Identification of Safety Practices for Evaluation

Search Strategy

The UCSF-Stanford Evidence-Based Practice Center Coordinating Team ("The Editors") provided general instructions to the teams of authors regarding search strategies for identifying safety practices for evaluation. As necessary, the Editors provided additional guidance and supplementary searches of the literature.

Search Strategy Recommended by Coordinating Team to Participating Reviewers

(a) *Electronic bibliographic databases*. All searches must include systematic searches of MEDLINE® and the Cochrane Library. For many topics it will be necessary to include other databases such as the Cumulative Index to Nursing & Allied Health (CINAHL), PsycLit (PsycINFO), the Institute for Scientific Information's *Science Citation Index Expanded*, *Social Sciences Citation Index*, *Arts & Humanities Citation Index*, INSPEC (physics, electronics and computing), and ABI/INFORM (business, management, finance, and economics).

(b) *Hand-searches of bibliographies of retrieved articles and tables of contents of key journals*.

(c) *Grey literature*. For many topics it will necessary to review the "grey literature," such as conference proceedings, institutional reports, doctoral theses, and manufacturers' reports.

(d) *Consultation with experts or workers in the field*.

To meet the early dissemination date mandated by AHRQ, the Editors did not require authors to search for non-English language articles or to use EMBASE. These were not specifically excluded, however, and authoring teams could include non-English language articles that addressed important aspects of a topic if they had translation services at their disposal. The Editors did not make recommendations on limiting database searches based on publication date. For this project it was particularly important to identify systematic reviews related to patient safety topics. Published strategies for retrieving systematic reviews have used proprietary MEDLINE® interfaces (e.g., OVID, SilverPlatter) that are not uniformly available. Moreover, the performance characteristics of these search strategies is unknown. Therefore, these strategies were not explicitly recommended. The Editors provided authors with a search algorithm (available upon request) that uses PubMed®, the freely available search interface from the National Library of Medicine, designed to retrieve systematic reviews with high sensitivity without overwhelming users with "false positive" hits. The Editors also performed independent searches of bibliographic databases and grey literature for selected topics. Concurrently, the EPC collaborated with NQF to solicit information about evidence-based practices from NQF members, and consulted with the project's Advisory Panel, whose members provided additional literature to review.

Inclusion and Exclusion Criteria

The EPC established criteria for selecting which of the identified safety practices warranted evaluation. The criteria address the applicability of the practice across a range of conditions or procedures and the available evidence of the practices' efficacy or effectiveness.

Inclusion/Exclusion Criteria for Practices

Inclusion Criteria

1. The practice can be applied in the hospital setting or at the interface between inpatient and outpatient settings AND can be applied to a broad range of healthcare conditions or procedures.
2. Evidence for the safety practice includes at least one study with a Level 3 or higher study design AND a Level 2 outcome measure. For practices not specifically related to diagnostic or therapeutic

interventions, a Level 3 outcome measure is adequate..

Exclusion Criterion

No study of the practice meets the methodologic criteria above. Practices that have only been studied outside the hospital setting or in patients with specific conditions or undergoing specific procedures were included if the authors and Editors agreed that the practices could reasonably be applied in the hospital setting and across a range of conditions or procedures. To increase the number of potentially promising safety practices adapted from outside the field of medicine, we included evidence from studies that used less rigorous measures of patient safety as long as the practices did not specifically relate to diagnostic or therapeutic interventions.

These criteria facilitated the inclusion of areas such as teamwork training and methods to improve information transfer. Each practice's level of evidence for efficacy or effectiveness was assessed in terms of study design and study outcomes . The Editors created the following hierarchies by modifying existing frameworks for evaluating evidence and incorporating recommendations from numerous other sources relevant to evidence synthesis.

Hierarchy of Study Designs

Level 1. *Randomized controlled trials*—includes quasi-randomized processes such as alternate allocation.

Level 2. *Non-randomized controlled trial*—a prospective (pre-planned) study, with predetermined eligibility criteria and outcome measures.

Level 3. *Observational studies with controls*—includes retrospective, interrupted time series (a change in trend attributable to the intervention), case-control studies, cohort studies with controls, and health services research that includes adjustment for likely confounding variables.

Level 4. *Observational studies without controls* (e.g., cohort studies without controls and case series)

Hierarchy of Outcome Measures

Level 1. *Clinical outcomes*—morbidity, mortality, adverse events.

Level 2. *Surrogate outcomes*—observed errors, intermediate outcomes (e.g., laboratory results) with well-established connections to the clinical outcomes of interest (usually adverse events).

Level 3. *Other measurable variables with an indirect or unestablished connection to the target safety outcome* (e.g., pre-test/post-test after an educational intervention, operator self-reports in different experimental situations).

Level 4. *No outcomes relevant to decreasing medical errors and/or adverse events* (e.g., study with patient satisfaction as only measured outcome; article describes an approach to detecting errors but reports no measured outcomes).

Implicit in this hierarchy of outcome measures is that surrogate or intermediate outcomes (Level 2) have an established relationship to the clinical outcomes (Level 1) of interest. Outcomes that are relevant to patient safety but have not been associated with morbidity or mortality were classified as Level 3.

Exceptions to EPC Criteria

Some safety practices did not meet the EPC inclusion criteria because of the paucity of evidence regarding efficacy or effectiveness, but were included in the Compendium because of their face validity (i.e., an informed reader might reasonably expect them to be evaluated). The reviews of these practices clearly identify the quality of evidence culled from medical and non-medical fields.

Evaluation of Safety Practices

For each practice, authors were instructed to research the literature for information on:

— Prevalence of the problem targeted by the practice.

— Severity of the problem targeted by the practice.

— The current utilisation of the practice.

— Evidence on efficacy and/or effectiveness of the practice.

— The practice's potential for harm.

— Data on cost if available.

— Implementation issues.

These elements were incorporated into a template in an effort to create as much uniformity across chapters as possible, especially given the widely disparate subject matter and quality of evidence. Since the amount of material for each practice was expected to, and did, vary substantially, the Editors provided general guidance on what was expected for each element, with particular detail devoted to the protocol for searching and reporting evidence related to efficacy and/or effectiveness of the practice.

The protocol outlined the search, the threshold for study inclusion, the elements to abstract from studies, and guidance on reporting information from each study. Authors were asked to review articles from their search to identify practices, and retain those with the better study designs. More focused searches were performed depending on the topic. The threshold for study inclusion related directly to study design. Authors were asked to use their judgment in deciding whether the evidence was sufficient at a given level of study design or whether the evidence from the next level needed to be reviewed.

At a minimum, the Editors suggested that there be at least 2 studies of adequate quality to justify excluding discussion of studies of lower level designs. Thus inclusion of 2 adequate clinical trials (Level 1 design) were necessary in order to exclude available evidence from prospective, non-randomized trials (Level 2) on the same topic. The Editors provided instructions for abstracting each article that met the inclusion criteria based on study design. For each study, a required set of 10 abstraction elements was specified. Authors received a detailed explanation of each required abstraction element, as well as complete abstraction examples for the 3 types of study design (Levels 1A, 1, and 3; Level 2 was not included since the information collected was same as Level 1). Research teams were encouraged to abstract any additional elements relevant to the specific subject area.

Ten Required Abstraction Elements

1. Bibliographic information according to *AMA Manual of Style*: title, authors, date of publication, source.
2. Level of study design (e.g., Level 1-3 for studies providing information for effectiveness; Level 4 if needed for relevant additional information) with descriptive material as follows:
3. Evidence-Based Review Methodology
   a. Identifiable description of methods indicating sources and methods of searching for articles.
   b. Stated inclusion and exclusion criteria for articles: yes/no.
   c. Scope of literature included in study.

For Level 1 or 2 Study Designs (Not Systematic Reviews)

a. Blinding: blinded, blinded (unclear), or unblinded
b. Describe comparability of groups at baseline—i.e., was distribution of potential confounders at baseline equal? If no, which confounders were not equal?
c. Loss to follow-up overall: percent of total study population lost to follow-up.

For Level 3 Study Design (Not Systematic Reviews)

a. Description of study design (e.g., case-control, interrupted time series).
b. Describe comparability of groups at baseline—i.e., was distribution of potential confounders at baseline equal? If no, which confounders were not equal?
c. Analysis includes adjustment for potential confounders: yes/no. If yes, adjusted for what confounders?
d. Description of intervention (as specific as possible).
e. Description of study population(s) and setting(s).
f. Level of relevant outcome measure(s) (e.g., Levels 1-4).
g. Description of relevant outcome measure(s).
h. Main Results: effect size with confidence intervals.
i. Information on unintended adverse (or beneficial) effects of practice.
j. Information on cost of practice.
k. Information on implementation of practice (information that might be of use in whether to and/or how to implement the practice—e.g., known barriers to implementation).

We present the salient elements of each included study (e.g., study design, population/setting, intervention details, results) in text or tabular form. In addition, we asked authors to highlight weaknesses and biases of studies where the interpretation of the results might be substantially affected. Authors were not asked to formally synthesize or combine (e.g., perform a meta-analysis) the evidence across studies for the Compendium.

REFERENCES

Apter AJ, Van Hoof TJ, Sherwin TE, Casey BA, Petrillo MK, Meehan TP. Assessing the quality of asthma care provided to Medicaid patients enrolled in managed care organisations in Connecticut. *Ann Allergy Asthma Immunol* 2001; 86:211-8.

Balas EA, Boren SA, Brown GD, Ewigman BG, Mitchell JA, Perkoff GT. Effect of physician profiling on utilization. Meta-analysis of randomized clinical trials. *J Gen Intern Med* 1996; 11:584-90.

Battles JB, Kaplan HS, Van der Schaaf TW, Shea CE. The attributes of medical event-reporting systems: experience with a prototype medical event-reporting system for transfusion medicine. *Arch Pathol Lab Med* 1998; 122:231-238.

Berman S. Identifying and addressing sentinel events: an Interview with Richard Croteau. *Jt Comm J Qual Improv* 1998; 24:426-434.

Bhasale A. The wrong diagnosis: identifying causes of potentially adverse events in general practice using incident monitoring. *Fam Pract* 1998; 15:308-318.

Bordley WC, Chelminski A, Margolis PA, Kraus R, Szilagyi PG, Vann JJ. The effect of audit and feedback on immunization delivery: a systematic review. *Am J Prev Med* 2000; 18:343-50.

Campbell CH Jr, Marum EM, Alwano-Edyegu MG, et al. The role of HIV counseling and testing in the developing world. AIDS Educ Prev 1997; 9(3Suppl):92-104.

Caplan RA, Posner KL, Cheney FW. Effect of outcome on physician judgments of appropriateness of care. *JAMA* 1991; 265:1957-1960.

Coyle S, Boruch R, Turner C, editors. Evaluating AIDS prevention programmes. Washington (DC): National Academy Press; 1991. p. 15-32.

Davis DA, Thomson MA, Oxman AD, Haynes RB. Changing physician performance. A systematic review of the effect of continuing medical education strategies. *JAMA* 1995; 274:700-5.

De Zoysa I, Philips KA, Kamenga MC, et al. Role of counseling and testing in changing risk behaviour in developing countries. AIDS 1995; 9(Suppl A):S95-S101.

Eagle CJ, Davies JM, Reason J. Accident analysis of large-scale technological disasters applied to an anaesthetic complication. *Can J Anaesth* 1992; 39:118-122.

Fernandes CM, Walker R, Price A, Marsden J, Haley L. Root cause analysis of laboratory delays to an emergency department. *J Emerg Med* 1997; 15:735-739.

Food and Drug Administration: Biological products; reporting of errors and accidents in manufacturing. *Fed Regist* 1997; 62:49642-49648.

Freemantle N, Harvey EL, Wolf F, Grimshaw JM, Grilli R, Bero LA. Printed educational materials: effects on professional practice and health care outcomes. In: *The Cochrane Library*, Issue 2, 2000. Oxford: Update Software.

Giacomini MK, Cook DJ. Users' guides to the medical literature: XXIII. Qualitative research in health care B. What are the results and how do they help me care for my patients? Evidence-Based Medicine Working Group. *JAMA* 2000; 284:478-482.

Grimshaw JM, Russell IT. Effect of clinical guidelines on medical practice: a systematic review of rigorous evaluations. *Lancet* 1993; 342:1317-22.

Higgins, DL, Galavotti, G, O'Reilly KR, et al. Evidence for effects of HIV antibody counseling and testing on risk behaviours. JAMA 1991; 266(17):2419-2429.

Hofer TP, Kerr EA. What is an error? *Eff Clin Pract* 2000; 3:261-269.

Ishikawa K. *What is total quality control? The Japanese way*. Englewood Cliffs, NJ: Prentice Hall. 1985.

Joint Commission on Accreditation of Healthcare Organisations. Sentinel Event Statistics. Available at: http://www.JCAHO.org. Accessed April 16, 2001.

Joint Commission on the Accreditation of Healthcare Organisations. Sentinel event policy and procedures. Available at: http://www.JCAHO.org/sentinel/se_pp.html. Accessed May 30, 2001.

Kaplan HS, Battles JB, Van der Schaaf TW, Shea CE, Mercer SQ. Identification and classification of the causes of events in transfusion medicine. *Transfusion* 1998; 38:1071-1081.

Leape LL, Bates DW, Cullen DJ, Cooper J, Demonaco HJ, Gallivan T, et al. Systems analysis of adverse drug events. ADE Prevention Study Group. *JAMA* 1995; 274:35-43.

Leape LL. Error in medicine. *JAMA* 1994; 272:1851-1857.

Moray N. Error reduction as a systems problem. In: Bogner M, editor. *Human error in medicine*. Hillsdale, NJ: Lawrence Erlbaum Associates. 1994.

Oxman AD, Thomson MA, Davis DA, Haynes RB. No magic bullets: a systematic review of 102 trials of interventions to improve professional practice. *CMAJ* 1995; 153:1423-31.

Perrow C. *Normal accidents: Living with High-Risk Technologies. With a New Afterword and a Postscript on the Y2K Problem*. Princeton, NJ: Princeton University Press. 1999.

Pope C, Mays N. Reaching the parts other methods cannot reach: an introduction to qualitative methods in health and health services research. *BMJ* 1995; 311:42-45.

Rabe KF, Vermeire PA, Soriano JB, Maier WC. Clinical management of asthma in 1999: the Asthma Insights and Reality in Europe (AIRE) study. *Eur Respir J* 2000; 16:802-7.

Rasmussen J. Human error and the problem of causality in analysis of accidents. *Philos Trans R Soc Lond B Biol Sci* 1990; 327:449-460.

Reason J. Human error: models and management. *BMJ* 2000; 320:768-770.

Reason JT. *Managing the Risks of Organisational Accidents*. Ashgate Publishing Company. 1997.

Rex JH, Turnbull JE, Allen SJ, Vande Voorde K, Luther K. Systematic root cause analysis of adverse drug events in a tertiary referral hospital. *Jt Comm J Qual Improv* 2000; 26:563-575.

Smith WR. Evidence for the effectiveness of techniques To change physician behaviour. *Chest* 2000; 118:8S-17S.

Szilagyi PG, Bordley C, Vann JC, Chelminski A, Kraus RM, Margolis PA, et al. Effect of patient reminder/recall interventions on immunization rates: A review. *JAMA* 2000; 284:1820-7.

Thomson O'Brien MA, Oxman AD, Davis DA, Haynes RB, Freemantle N, Harvey EL. Audit and feedback: effects on professional practice and health care outcomes. In: *The Cochrane Library*, Issue 2, 2000:Oxford: Update Software.

Thomson O'Brien MA, Oxman AD, Davis DA, Haynes RB, Freemantle N, Harvey EL. Audit and feedback versus alternative strategies: effects on professional practice and health care outcomes. In: *The Cochrane Library*, Issue 2, 2000. Oxford: Update Software.

Thomson O'Brien MA, Oxman AD, Davis DA, Haynes RB, Freemantle N, Harvey EL. Educational outreach visits: effects on professional practice and health care outcomes. In: *The Cochrane Library*, Issue 2, 2000. Oxford: Update Software.

Thomson O'Brien MA, Oxman AD, Haynes RB, Davis DA, Freemantle N, Harvey EL. Local opinion leaders: effects on professional practice and health care outcomes. In: *The Cochrane Library*, Issue 2, 2000. Oxford: Update Software..

Troidl H. Disasters of endoscopic surgery and how to avoid them: error analysis. *World J Surg* 1999; 23:846-855.

Bibliography

Allan EL, Barker KN. Fundamentals of medication error research. *Am J Hosp Pharm* 1990; 47:555-571.

Bailey KR. Generalizing the results of randomized clinical trials. *Control Clin Trials* 1994; 15:15-23.

Barker KN, Pearson RE, Hepler CD, Smith WE, Pappas CA. Effect of an automated bedside dispensing machine on medication errors. *Am J Hosp Pharm* 1984; 41:1352-1358.

Bates DW, Boyle DL, Vander Vliet MB, Schneider J, Leape L. Relationship between medication errors and adverse drug events. *J Gen Intern Med* 1995; 10:199-205.

Bates DW, Cullen DJ, Laird N, Petersen LA, Small SD, Servi D, et al. Incidence of adverse drug events and potential adverse drug events: Implications for prevention. *JAMA* 1995; 274:29-34.

Benson K, Hartz AJ. A comparison of observational studies and randomized, controlled trials. *N Engl J Med* 2000; 342:1878-1886.

Borel JM, Rascati KL. Effect of an automated, nursing unit-based drug-dispensing device on medication errors. *Am J Health Syst Pharm* 1995; 52:1875-1879.

Bucher HC, Guyatt GH, Cook DJ, Holbrook A, McAlister FA. Users' guides to the medical literature: XIX. Applying clinical trial results. A. How to use an article measuring the effect of an intervention on surrogate end points.

Evidence-Based Medicine Working Group. *JAMA* 1999; 282:771-778.

Classen DC, Pestotnik SL, Evans RS, Lloyd JF, Burke JP. Adverse drug events in hospitalized patients. Excess length of stay, extra costs, and attributable mortality. *JAMA* 1997; 277:301-306.

Concato J, Shah N, Horwitz RI. Randomized, controlled trials, observational studies, and the hierarchy of research designs. *N Engl J Med* 2000; 342:1887-1892.

Cullen DJ, Sweitzer BJ, Bates DW, Burdick E, Edmondson A, Leape LL. Preventable adverse drug events in hospitalized patients: a comparative study of intensive care and general care units. *Crit Care Med* 1997; 25:1289-1297.

Dean B, Barber N. Validity and reliability of observational methods for studying medication administration errors. *Am J Health Syst Pharm* 2001; 58:54-59.

Dean BS, Allan EL, Barber ND, Barker KN. Comparison of medication errors in an American and British hospital. *Am J Health Syst Pharm* 1995; 52:2543-2549.

Facchinetti NJ, Campbell GM, Jones DP. Evaluating dispensing error detection rates in a hospital pharmacy. *Med Care* 1999; 37:39-43.

Felkey BG, Barker KN. Technology and automation in pharmaceutical care. *J Am Pharm Assoc (Wash)* 1996; NS36:309-314.

Glanville J, Lefebvre C. Identifying systematic reviews: key resources. *ACP J Club* 2000; 132:A11-A12.

Gotzsche PC, Liberati A, Torri V, Rossetti L. Beware of surrogate outcome measures. *Int J Technol Assess Health Care* 1996; 12:238-246.

Guerrero RM, Nickman NA, Jorgenson JA. Work activities

before and after implementation of an automated dispensing system. *Am J Health Syst Pharm* 1996; 53:548-554.

Guyatt G, Schunemann H, Cook D, Jaeschke R, Pauker S, Bucher H. Grades of recommendation for antithrombotic agents. *Chest* 2001; 119:3S-7S.

Guyatt GH, Sackett DL, Sinclair JC, Hayward R, Cook DJ, Cook RJ. Users' guides to the medical literature. IX. A method for grading health care recommendations. Evidence-Based Medicine Working Group. *JAMA* 1995; 274:1800-1804.

Guyatt GH, Tugwell PX, Feeny DH, Drummond MF, Haynes RB. The role of before-after studies of therapeutic impact in the evaluation of diagnostic technologies. *J Chronic Dis* 1986; 39:295-304.

Harris RP, Helfand M, Woolf SH, Lohr KN, Mulrow CD, Teutsch SM, et al. Current methods of the U.S. Preventive Services Task Force. A review of the process. *Am J Prev Med* 2001; 20:21-35.

Hunt DL, McKibbon KA. Locating and appraising systematic reviews. *Ann Intern Med* 1997; 126:532-538.

Jadad AR, Cook DJ, Browman GP. A guide to interpreting discordant systematic reviews. *CMAJ* 1997; 156:1411-1416.

Juni P, Witschi A, Bloch R, Egger M. The hazards of scoring the quality of clinical trials for meta-analysis. *JAMA* 1999; 282:1054-1060.

Klein EG, Santora JA, Pascale PM, Kitrenos JG. Medication cart-filling time, accuracy, and cost with an automated dispensing system. *Am J Hosp Pharm* 1994; 51:1193-1196.

Levine M, Walter S, Lee H, Haines T, Holbrook A, Moyer V.

Users' guides to the medical literature. IV. How to use an article about harm. Evidence-Based Medicine Working Group. *JAMA* 1994; 271:1615-1619.

McAuley L, Pham B, Tugwell P, Moher D. Does the inclusion of grey literature influence estimates of intervention effectiveness reported in meta-analyses? *Lancet* 2000; 356:1228-1231.

McKee M, Britton A, Black N, McPherson K, Sanderson C, Bain C. Methods in health services research. Interpreting the evidence: choosing between randomised and non-randomised studies. *BMJ* 1999; 319:312-315.

Moher D, Jadad AR, Tugwell P. Assessing the quality of randomized controlled trials. Current issues and future directions. *Int J Technol Assess Health Care* 1996; 12:195-208.

Muir Gray JA, Haynes RB, Sackett DL, Cook DJ, Guyatt GH. Transferring evidence from research into practice: 3. Developing evidence-based clinical policy. *ACP J Club* 1997; 126:A14-A16.

Mulrow C, Langhorne P, Grimshaw J. Integrating heterogeneous pieces of evidence in systematic reviews. *Ann Intern Med* 1997; 127:989-995.

Murray MD. Information technology: the infrastructure for improvements to the medication-use process. *Am J Health Syst Pharm* 2000; 57:565-571.

Naylor CD, Guyatt GH. Users' guides to the medical literature. X. How to use an article reporting variations in the outcomes of health services. The Evidence-Based Medicine Working Group. *JAMA* 1996; 275:554-558.

Omnicell Automated Systems. Omnicell Homepage. Available at: http://www.omnicell.com. Accessed May 28, 2001.

Oxman AD, Cook DJ, Guyatt GH. Users' guides to the

medical literature. VI. How to use an overview. Evidence-Based Medicine Working Group. *JAMA* 1994; 272:1367-1371.

Perini VJ, Vermeulen LC, Jr. Comparison of automated medication-management systems. *Am J Hosp Pharm* 1994; 51:1883-1891.

Ringold DJ, Santell JP, Schneider PJ. ASHP national survey of pharmacy practice in acute care settings: dispensing and administration—1999. *Am J Health Syst Pharm* 2000; 57:1759-1775.

Schwarz HO, Brodowy BA. Implementation and evaluation of an automated dispensing system. *Am J Health Syst Pharm* 1995; 52:823-828.

Shirley KL. Effect of an automated dispensing system on medication administration time. *Am J Health Syst Pharm* 1999; 56:1542-1545.

Shojania KG, Bero L. Taking advantage of the explosion of systematic reviews: an efficient MEDLINE search strategy. *Eff Clin Pract* 2001; 4: in press.

Stroup DF, Berlin JA, Morton SC, Olkin I, Williamson GD, Rennie D, et al. Meta-analysis of observational studies in epidemiology: a proposal for reporting. Meta-analysis Of Observational Studies in Epidemiology (MOOSE) group. *JAMA* 2000; 283:2008-2012.

Thurfjell E, Thurfjell MG, Egge E, Bjurstam N. Sensitivity and specificity of computer-assisted breast cancer detection in mammography screening. *Acta Radiol* 1998; 39:384-388.

Tissot E, Cornette C, Demoly P, Jacquet M, Barale F, Capellier G. Medication errors at the administration stage in an intensive care unit. *Intensive Care Med* 1999; 25:353-3359.

Index

Q

R

S

T

U

W

Y